‘This book is a marvellous interdisciplinary synthesis, grounded in case examples and at once critical and constructive. As such, it is both instructive for policy practitioners as well as moving the scholarship of the field forward.’ – *Vivian Lin, Professor of Public Health, La Trobe University, Australia*

‘This is essential reading for anybody working on the smarter use of evidence by government. It catalogues the many biases twisting how research is used by policymakers. It also addresses a vital challenge in our sector – a lack of legitimacy. As well as the academic rigour of this book, there are practical tips on what we can do about these problems, and lessons from across the globe showing where we get it wrong – and how we might get it right.’ – *Jonathan Breckon, Head of the Alliance for Useful Evidence, UK*

‘This important book goes well beyond standard analyses of evidence informed policy with detailed discussions of the politics of evidence and the political origins (and the cognitive psychology) of bias in the use of research evidence. It addresses a core and often overlooked issue of the governance of evidence use – including the need to consider the institutions and processes in place that can enable the appropriate use of evidence in decision making. This book will be a pretty essential read for anyone concerned with the policy, practice or study of using research to inform decision making.’ – *David Gough, Professor of Evidence Informed Policy and Practice, Director of the EPPI-Centre, University College London, UK*

The Politics of Evidence

There has been an enormous increase in interest in the use of evidence for public policymaking, but the vast majority of work on the subject has failed to engage with the political nature of decision making and how this influences the ways in which evidence will be used (or misused) within political areas. This book provides new insights into the nature of political bias with regards to evidence and critically considers what an 'improved' use of evidence would look like from a policymaking perspective.

Part I describes the great potential for evidence to help achieve social goals, as well as the challenges raised by the political nature of policymaking. It explores the concern of evidence advocates that political interests drive the misuse or manipulation of evidence, as well as counter-concerns of critical policy scholars about how appeals to 'evidence-based policy' can depoliticise political debates. Both concerns reflect forms of *bias* – the first representing *technical bias*, whereby evidence use violates principles of scientific best practice, and the second representing *issue bias* in how appeals to evidence can shift political debates to particular questions or marginalise policy-relevant social concerns.

Part II then draws on the fields of policy studies and cognitive psychology to understand the origins and mechanisms of both forms of bias in relation to political interests and values. It illustrates how such biases are not only common, but can be much more predictable once we recognise their origins and manifestations in policy arenas.

Finally, Part III discusses ways to move forward for those seeking to improve the use of evidence in public policymaking. It explores what constitutes 'good evidence for policy', as well as the 'good use of evidence' within policy processes, and considers how to build evidence-advisory institutions that embed key principles of both scientific good practice and democratic representation. Taken as a whole, the approach promoted is termed the 'good governance of evidence' – a concept that represents the use of rigorous, systematic and technically valid pieces of evidence within decision-making processes that are representative of, and accountable to, populations served.

Justin Parkhurst is an Associate Professor at the London School of Economics and Political Science's Department of Social Policy. This book was written while he was previously Senior Lecturer at the London School of Hygiene and Tropical Medicine's Department of Global Health and Development.

Routledge Studies in Governance and Public Policy

16 **Democratic Governance and Social Entrepreneurship**
Civic participation and the future of democracy
Denise M. Horn

17 **Health Care Policy and Opinion in the United States and Canada**
Richard Nadeau, Éric Bélanger, François Pétry, Stuart Soroka, Antonia Maioni

18 **Inclusive Growth, Development and Welfare Policy**
A Critical Assessment
Edited by Reza Hasmath

19 **The New and Changing Transatlanticism**
Politics and Policy Perspectives
Edited by Laurie Buonanno Natalia Cuglesan and Keith Henderson

20 **Childhood Citizenship, Governance and Policy**
The politics of becoming adult
Sana Nakata

21 **The Idea of Good Governance and the Politics of the Global South**
An Analysis of its Effects
Haroon A. Khan

22 **Interpreting Governance, High Politics and Public Policy**
Essays commemorating Interpreting British Governance
Edited by Nick Turnbull

23 **Political Engagement of the Young in Europe**
Youth in the crucible
Edited by Peter Thijssen, Jessy Siongers, Jeroen Van Laer, Jacques Haers and Sara Mels

24 **Rethinking Governance**
Ruling, rationalities and resistance
Edited by Mark Bevir and R. A. W. Rhodes

25 **Governmentality after Neoliberalism**
Edited by Mark Bevir

26 **Transformational Public Policy**
A new strategy for coping with uncertainty and risk
Mark Matthews

27 **The Public Legitimacy of Minority Claims**
A Central/Eastern European Perspective
Plamen Makariev

The Politics of Evidence

From evidence-based policy to the good governance of evidence

Justin Parkhurst

Routledge
Taylor & Francis Group
LONDON AND NEW YORK

First published 2017
by Routledge

2 Park Square, Milton Park, Abingdon, Oxfordshire OX14 4RN
711 Third Avenue, New York, NY 10017

Routledge is an imprint of the Taylor & Francis Group, an informa business

First issued in paperback 2017

British Library Cataloguing in Publication Data
A catalogue record for this book is available from the British Library

Library of Congress Cataloging in Publication Data
Names: Parkhurst, Justin O., author.
Title: The politics of evidence : from evidence-based policy to the good governance of evidence / Justin Parkhurst.
Description: Abingdon, Oxon ; New York, NY : Routledge, 2017. | Includes bibliographical references and index.
Identifiers: LCCN 2016022525| ISBN 9781138939400 (hardback) | ISBN 9781315675008 (ebook)
Subjects: LCSH: Policy sciences. | Research—Evaluation. | Social policy.
Classification: LCC H97 .P3725 2017 | DDC 320.6—dc23
LC record available at https://lccn.loc.gov/2016022525

ISBN: 978-1-138-93940-0 (hbk)
ISBN: 978-1-138-57038-2 (pbk)

Typeset in Times New Roman
by Swales & Willis Ltd, Exeter, Devon, UK

For Skye and Rae

Contents

Figures

Tables

Boxes

Acknowledgements

This work was supported by a grant from the European Research Council (GRIP-Health: Getting Research into Policy in Health, grant #282118). I would like to thank the London School of Hygiene and Tropical Medicine, as well as my colleagues there for their numerous insights and discussions that helped to inform the ideas in this book. In particular, I would like to acknowledge the work of those individuals who worked within the GRIP-Health programme – Sudeepa Abeysinghe, Arturo Alvarez-Rosete, Stefanie Ettelt, Benjamin Hawkins, Marco Liverani, Fiona Marquet, Elisa Vecchione, Ioana Vlad and Helen Walls – as well as Eleanor Hutchinson, who contributed to the programme's initial ideas. I would also like to thank Rakesh Narayana for his early research assistance and Siobhan Leir for assistance in proofreading this book. I am furthermore incredibly grateful to Louise Shaxson for reviewing the final manuscript at short notice.

Figure 3.1 was reproduced freely with thanks to Bobby Henderson. Chapter 6 expands on an earlier working paper written with Sudeepa Abeysinghe in 2013, subsequently published in 2016. Elements of Chapter 7, including the importance of the legitimacy of the process by which evidence is used, were inspired by doctoral findings of Bianca D'Souza, as well as doctoral work of David Chilongozi. The concept of the 'good governance of evidence' and the framework developed in Chapter 8 has its origins in many discussions and outputs related to the GRIP-Health research programme. Early programme team discussions identified good governance as a critical lens to consider how to judge improved evidence-use. A funding proposal developed with Kalipso Chalkidou in 2013 further used the term the 'good governance of evidence', and elaborated upon the idea of making incremental changes within national programmes guided by key principles of good evidentiary practice as a strategy for capacity building (ideas incorporated into Chapter 8). An initial conceptual framework on the good governance of evidence was also developed in a paper published with Benjamin Hawkins in 2015, which is expanded upon and developed further in this book's final chapter.

My final and deepest thanks, however, go to my wife and family for their support during the writing of this book.

Part I

Evidence-based policymaking

Opportunities and challenges

1 Introduction

Evidence matters (three examples)

- For most of the second half of the twentieth century, new parents were advised by medical professionals to place babies to sleep on their fronts – with advocates such as the popular paediatrician Dr Benjamin Spock explaining this could reduce the risk of infants choking in their sleep if they were to vomit (Howick 2011). This practice continued for decades while empirical studies were slowly accumulating evidence that, in fact, babies left to sleep on their fronts might be at higher risk of sudden infant death syndrome (SIDS) than back-sleepers. Finally, in 2005, a systematic review of the literature was published which identified the relative risk of SIDS to be nearly three times *higher* for front-sleepers. The authors of the review argued that, had a more rigorous review of evidence been done in the 1970s, this 'might have prevented over 10,000 infant deaths in the UK and at least 50,000 in Europe, the USA, and Australasia' (Gilbert et al. 2005, p. 874).
- In the 1970s and 1980s, the oil company Exxon was undertaking extensive research on the effect of burning fossil fuels on the environment. According to a recently published investigation of the company's internal documents, it was found that as early as 1977, Exxon was aware that carbon dioxide emissions from fossil fuel use could lead to significant and potentially harmful climate change (Banerjee, Song and Hasemyer 2015). According to the investigators, rather than disseminating these findings, the company appeared to promote misinformation on the topic in the decades that followed, claiming that climate change science was 'still controversial' and funding organisations like the 'Global Climate Coalition' that disputed the science of climate change (Banerjee, Song and Hasemyer 2015; Hall 2015). Exxon's response to the accusations was to argue that the company has had 'a continuous and uninterrupted commitment to climate change research' (Onthemedia 2015).
- In January, 2003, just a few months before the US sent military forces into Iraq, US President George W. Bush built his case for invasion in his annual 'State of the Union' address. In the speech, he presented evidence that many took to be illustrative of a compelling and imminent security risk posed by the Iraqi regime, including a particularly powerful 16-word statement that:

'The British government has learned that Saddam Hussein recently sought significant quantities of uranium from Africa.'[1] President Bush's case for war was particularly controversial, however, with accusations soon being made that the administration misled the public through inaccurate, or potentially even deceptive, uses of evidence (cf. Hartnett and Stengrim 2004; Jamieson 2007; Pfiffner 2004). Indeed, only six months after President Bush made the statement above, George Tenet, the Director of the CIA, stated that: 'These 16 words [about uranium] should never have been included in the text written for the president' (Tenet 2003).

Evidence *matters* for public policymaking. Advocates of greater evidence utilisation commonly point to examples like the first one given above to show how more rigorous or more widespread use of evidence could avoid unnecessary harms and help achieve important social policy goals. Evidence tells us 'what works'. Yet these individuals also particularly fear and lament what is demonstrated in the other two cases – the potential for cherry-picking, obfuscation or manipulation of pieces of evidence, done to serve political goals. The *misuse of evidence* matters as well and, for evidence champions, the way to address these concerns has been through the use of *evidence-based policymaking* (EBP), in which policy decisions are expected to follow from rigorous and accurate uses of scientific evidence.

Such calls for policies to be evidence-based have proliferated so widely in the past few decades as to become a movement unto itself, with calls for increased EBP heard within government bureaucracies, academic institutions and the media alike. We also see the embrace of so-called 'hierarchies of evidence', which have been seen as ways to rank or prioritise different types of evidence for policy consideration (Nutley, Powell and Davies 2013). These ideas have further led to EBP becoming an expectation against which political actors can be judged, as seen when criticism has been levelled against governments in cases such as the following: the Canadian government pursuing criminal justice policies based on an 'emotionally satisfying tough stance' instead of an EBP (Adams 2015); the Indian government establishing a new Ministry of Yoga without evidence of effectiveness (Kumar 2014); or the British government pursuing immigration restrictions based on public perceptions of immigrants abusing the benefits system rather than evidence showing migrants are less likely to claim benefits than nationals (Partos 2014).

We can also see an enormously wide range of policy decisions where calls are made to be 'evidence-based'. Examples include the American Medical Association (AMA) arguing that: 'Laws that regulate abortion should be evidence-based and designed to improve women's health' (Barnes 2016), the South African government pursuing an 'evidence-based' approach to its employment tax policy, or a *British Medical Journal* commentary arguing that: 'Dog ownership has unknown risks but known health benefits: we need evidence based policy' (Orritt 2014).

1 Transcript available from: http://www.washingtonpost.com/wp-srv/onpolitics/transcripts/bushtext_012803.html.

Critical voices

Despite this seeming ubiquity of the concept, there is a growing body of academic writing that is highly critical of the idea that social policies can somehow simply be 'based' on evidence alone. Authors informed by the policy sciences have long recognised that public policymaking is not the same thing as technical decision making. Rather, policymaking typically involves trade-offs between multiple competing social values, with only a very small proportion of policy decisions simply concerned with technical evidence of the effects of interventions (Weiss 1979; Lin 2003; Russell et al. 2008). As early as the 1970s, Rittel and Webber declared that 'The search for scientific bases for confronting problems of social policy is bound to fail' (1973, p. 155), with the authors coining the term 'wicked problems' to distinguish what makes many social policy decisions particularly hard to solve. They explain that:

> in a pluralistic society there is nothing like the undisputable public good; there is no objective definition of equity; policies that respond to social problems cannot be meaningfully correct or false; and it makes no sense to talk about 'optimal solutions' to social problems unless severe qualifications are imposed first. Even worse, there are no 'solutions' in the sense of definitive and objective answers.
>
> (Ibid.)

Given this fundamentally contested nature of most public policy concerns, the use of evidence *for policy* has been described as 'qualitatively different' (Black 2001) than its use in technical decision-making arenas (such as clinical medicine). Indeed, over half a century ago, political theorists noted that policymaking centrally involves decisions about what a good society should look like – questions that science alone cannot answer (Brecht 1959). As such, calls for policy to simply be 'evidence-based' have been described as 'naïve rationality' – incorrectly assuming that policymaking is merely an exercise in 'decision science', when the policy process is, instead, a 'struggle over ideas and values' (Russell et al. 2008, p. 40). As such, some have dismissed the entire idea of EBP as a 'myth' (Hammersley 2013) – nothing more than a 'technocratic wish in a political world' (Lewis 2003, p. 250).

These perspectives raise important challenges to many of the contemporary calls for public policy decisions to be 'evidence-based'. This is particularly true for highly contested issues where multiple social values and concerns are at stake. The AMA's call for abortion policy to be 'evidence-based' to improve women's health, for example, appears to show a remarkable lack of recognition of the actual terms of the abortion debate in America. The debate over abortion in the US is not over whether or not it leads to health harms for women; rather, it is primarily discussed in terms of *rights* – rights of women over their bodies or rights of the unborn. Opponents to abortion do not oppose it because they think making it illegal will improve women's health – they oppose it because they believe it to be fundamentally wrong to terminate pregnancies. Similarly, many supporters of abortion would likely continue to support it as a right even if evidence existed that found the procedure to be potentially harmful from a health perspective. What an 'evidence-based' abortion policy would be therefore depends on the social values or concerns one holds to be important – for the AMA, it might be health harms, but for many stakeholders, health is not the main issue.

A call for policies on dog ownership to be 'evidence-based' similarly shows how far the EBP concept has been stretched and how flimsy it can be when it is subject to some basic questioning. The author of that commentary argues that we need EBP based on the risks and health benefits involved. Yet what might such evidence look like? And would it naturally lead to an obvious policy choice? In the article, the risks are presented as the rare (but often severe) attacks by dogs on members of the public, while the benefits reflect psychological well-being of dog owners. But even knowing this information, does an obvious 'evidence-based policy' emerge? Would the risk of bites lead to a policy to ban dogs? To restrict their location? To require muzzles? To require licences? To require training? The evidence provided cannot decide this on its own. We can also ask if bites and psychological benefits are the only pieces of evidence that are relevant for an 'evidence-based' dog ownership policy. Many dog owners would say they love their pets regardless of any health benefits. Should some assessment of this be included as evidence as well? What about the carbon footprint of owning a dog, the stress levels on local cats or the noise complaints of neighbours? There is no obvious indication of *which* evidence is the *right* evidence on which to base such policy and, indeed, there is likely to be disagreement over the relevance or importance of different social policy concerns. Yet what is particularly concerning is that such questions are typically not even asked within many modern calls for public policies to be 'evidence-based'.

A politically informed perspective, then, must begin from a recognition that policies typically involve multiple social concerns, and there can be different evidence bases relevant to each one. Many advocates of evidence see the embrace of evidence (particularly scientific evidence) as a means to transcend the corrupting nature of politics – as a means to avoid cases like those at the start of this chapter where political influence led to the misuse of evidence. Yet others have raised concern about how the EBP language can, in fact, obscure the relevant social values at stake when these should instead be transparent. Wesselink et al., for instance, explain that: 'Overt deference to EBP does not remove the need for political reasoning; rather politics is introduced "through the back door" through debates on what is valid evidence rather than on what values should prevail' (Wesselink, Colebatch, and Pearce 2014, p. 341).

In other words, rather than being *apolitical*, the appeal to evidence, or to particular forms of evidence, can be *decidedly political* by promoting a de facto choice amongst competing values. The politics comes in 'through the back door' by giving political priority to those things which have been measured or those things which are conducive to measuring (Barnes and Parkhurst 2014;

Parkhurst and Abeysinghe 2016). Looking again at the AMA's brief to the Supreme Court from this perspective, we can see that it is making a decidedly political argument couched in the language of EBP – specifically, the AMA is arguing that the basis of abortion laws should be the principle of medical harms to women. Yet while this may be an important social concern and the one on which we have the clearest quantitative evidence, others in the abortion debates may disagree that this evidence base means it is *most* relevant or the *only* issue on which such laws should be based.

Two (quite different) forms of bias

The competing perspectives on EBP have, at times, deeply divided individuals writing on the subject. Parsons explains that 'there are profound ontological, epistemological and methodological differences between those who believe in [EBP] and those who have doubts as to its feasibility or the values it embodies' (2002, p. 45). Some have even referred to the debates between camps as a 'paradigm war' waged between 'positivist empiricists' on the one hand and 'critical interpretevists' on the other (Greenhalgh and Russell 2009).

The critical perspective therefore sees EBP as failing to address the realities of policymaking, with some seeing the term as nothing more than empty rhetoric (cf. Hammersley 2005, 2013). For evidence champions, the response to these arguments has been to dismiss them as overly theoretical and to reiterate the point that evidence-based decisions can ensure that we are doing more good than harm, pointing to those clear cases where evidence use 'works in practice' and has improved outcomes or even saved lives (cf. Chalmers 2005). Others who do not fall into one camp or the other are often left in the middle, questioning whether the realities of policymaking mean that we cannot say *anything* about how to improve evidence use, even if we wish to achieve social goals more efficiently.

Moving beyond this seeming impasse is possible, but it requires recognising that both perspectives have valid and useful insights to provide. Progress requires neither a blind embrace of EBP nor a complete rejection of it as a concept. Instead, this book attempts to move these debates forward by recognition that a key problem for both sides lies in the *politics of evidence*, but their normative concerns are very different in nature. For champions of evidence, there is a problem with the *politicisation of science* – and the ways that political interests appear to drive the misuse, manipulation, or cherry picking of evidence to promote political interests (Pielke 2002; Wise 2006). This can be otherwise be defined as a concern over *technical bias* in the use of evidence – evidence utilisation that does not follow principles of scientific best practice (which can include invalid uses of individual pieces of evidence, as well failing to systematically include all the relevant evidence that best answers a particular question) and which therefore leads to poorer policy outcomes than would otherwise be possible. The critical policy perspective, on the other hand, points to the problems caused by the *depoliticisation of politics* – in particular the ways in which social values can be obscured or marginalised through the promotion of certain forms or bodies of evidence. This is also a form of bias, but can alternatively be termed *issue bias* to capture how evidence utilisation can shift the political debate to particular questions or concerns in a non-transparent way. The first form of bias broadly reflects the value of scientific fidelity, while the second broadly reflects the value of democratic representation.

Defined as such, it becomes clearer that these positions need not be seen as mutually exclusive when they are considered based on their normative rather than their epistemological differences. In this way, this book takes a decidedly pragmatic approach, recognising that both sets of values are important goals to pursue within efforts to improve the use of evidence for policymaking. It therefore looks to identify ways to address both sets of concerns given the political realities of policy processes. From this perspective, however, the goal of improving evidence use can no longer be seen as a simple question of doing 'what works'. Addressing both sets of issues – and reducing instances or the impact of both technical and issue bias – requires moving beyond past efforts to simply call for more EBP, greater evidence 'uptake' or the blind application of evidence hierarchies. Rather, it demands deeper investigation of the political origins of bias to help guide efforts to avoid bias or mitigate its impact. Furthermore, an explicit desire to improve the use of evidence in policy will require the establishment of new principles of what would constitute *good evidence to inform policy*, as well as considering what constitutes the *good use of evidence* within a policy process.

This approach does not reject the importance of evidence. It accepts that there can indeed be more or less technically accurate uses of evidence. Pieces of evidence can be manipulated or they can be presented faithfully to their findings. Bodies of evidence can be cherry-picked or they can be reviewed systematically. Research designs can be valid and rigorous or they can be created on flawed scientific foundations to achieve a pre-desired conclusion. These are all important to address if evidence is to have a future in informing policymaking. Yet this book also understands that policymaking fundamentally involves competition between multiple social goals and the pursuit of social values. As such, there are additional concerns that this brings to the table, such as which social interests are addressed by evidence in the first place, whether these interests are more or less transparent in policy debates, or if they are pursued through more or less representative processes.

This book argues that efforts to improve evidence use will ultimately require building systems that work to embed key normative principles about evidence utilisation into policy processes – systems that can be said to *govern* the use of evidence within policymaking. Therefore, in order to move the EBP field forward, it is necessary to consider how to establish *evidence advisory systems* that promote the *good governance of evidence* – working to ensure that rigorous, systematic and technically valid pieces of evidence are used within decision-making processes that are inclusive of, representative of and accountable to the multiple social interests of the population served.

From EBP to the good governance of evidence

Achieving this requires embracing the political nature of policymaking head-on. This book therefore applies a decidedly political perspective (informed by the academic fields of public policy and policy studies in particular) that highlights two key issues about the nature of public policymaking. The first is to recognise that policy decisions are *political* because they involve trade-offs between multiple competing interests, as noted above. Politics is, as Lasswell famously described in the 1930s, about 'who gets what, when, and how' (Lasswell 1990 [1936]). This is what particularly distinguishes policy decisions from technical exercises weighing up data on a single agreed outcome. Instead, it is common, or indeed the norm, for there to be disagreements in society about which social outcomes are important or how to value different arrangements of social outcomes.

It is worth noting that from this perspective, evidence is not irrelevant. Evidence serves as a tool of measurement. It can help identify who will benefit from different choices or how much different benefits will accrue to different groups. But there will also be a fundamental need to have transparency over the different social concerns at stake, and recognition of the contestation over how to value different outcomes. Evidence cannot tell us which is the *right* choice between different arrangements of benefits or which social outcomes should be pursued over others. Such decisions must be made on the basis of some formal consideration of social values, which modern democratic principles would argue needs to be done in transparent and accountable ways that serve to represent the public.

The second key approach that the political perspective of this book utilises is the recognition that political decisions take place within contextually specific institutional structures that direct, shape or constrain the range of possible policy choices and outcomes. The field of policy studies known as *institutionalism* has developed out of a recognition that political institutional arrangements greatly affect policy processes and outcomes, including dictating which issues are considered by decision makers, whose interests are represented or the steps and processes through which decisions can or cannot be made (Rothstein 1996; Peters 2005; Lowndes 2010). All public policy decisions can therefore be seen to be made within some form of institutional arrangements, with evidence-informed policy decisions being no exception.

These insights provide the basic framework used by this book to address the politics of evidence, moving from the idea of 'evidence-based policy' and a depoliticised and decontextualised search for 'what works' to instead consider how to establish the good governance of evidence. The first section of the book addresses some of the principle issues covered. Chapter 2 explores the need and great potential of evidence use in public policymaking in more depth. It reflects on the origins of the modern EBP concept in the field of evidence-based medicine, the efforts made to date to promote evidence use through so-called 'knowledge transfer' efforts, and the limitations these approaches face given the political nature of policymaking. It reiterates the need for a political approach that considers multiple competing values as well as the political institutional context in which decision making takes place, particularly exploring *what's wrong* with the simple idea of doing *what works* from a policy perspective.

Part II of the book addresses the 'politics of evidence' by exploring the political origins of evidentiary bias in particular. Chapter 3 discusses the two forms of bias – technical bias and issue bias – in greater depth to construct a framework on the multiple politics of evidence, reflecting on empirical examples of how bias may manifest within the creation, selection or interpretation of evidence. Chapter 4 then considers what is termed the 'overt politics of evidence' to capture bias that derives from politically motivated groups pursuing their interests in a competitive political arena. It notes that if political debate is about competition and contestation, then there is no reason to believe that adherence to scientific good practice will necessarily be a priority for those involved. The chapter provides a number of examples to reflect on how the competitive nature of policymaking can generate technical and issue bias, such as through pressure to show results, efforts to undermine science or appeals to 'evidence' as a purely rhetorical strategy to gain support. The chapter argues that understanding the nature of political competition should make such forms of bias not only more evident, but also more predictable.

Chapter 5 then follows with another exploration of the political origins of bias. Yet while Chapter 4 discussed what was termed the 'overt politics of evidence' arising from the direct pursuit of competing interests, Chapter 5 explores what is termed the 'subtle politics of evidence' that can arise through unconscious processes. The chapter draws on cognitive psychological research to provide a new perspective on how social values contribute to both technical and issue bias, providing a range of examples of how such processes affect politicians, laypersons and technical experts alike. The chapter concludes by developing a 'cognitive political model' of evidentiary bias that maps out how key features of policy debates – such as their complexity, their contestation or their polarisation – can generate both technical and issue bias through differing mechanisms (both overt and subtle).

The final part of the book then turns towards the questions of how to improve the use of evidence, given our greater understanding of the origins and manifestations of technical and issue bias. It argues that this requires the establishment of new principles on which to guide such efforts. Chapter 6 begins this by exploring what constitutes 'good evidence for policy' in order to move beyond technical hierarchies that may be insufficient or inappropriately applied from a policy perspective. Instead, it draws on a set of academic disciplines (political studies, the sociology of knowledge and the philosophy of science) to construct a 'framework of appropriateness' through which to consider policy relevant evidence (based on an earlier discussion in Parkhurst and Abeysinghe (2016)). Within this framework, *appropriate evidence* is identified as that which speaks to the multiple social concerns at stake in a policy decision, which is constructed in the ways that are most useful to achieve policy goals, and which is applicable in the local policy context. *Good evidence for policy* is subsequently defined as evidence which is appropriate according to these conditions and which further meets high quality standards from a scientific perspective.

Chapter 7 then addresses the question of what constitutions the *good use of evidence* from a policy perspective. Rather than an exploration of scientific principles, however, this chapter particularly engages with democratic theory to reflect on what is needed in order for policy decision processes – including those involving evidence use – to be seen as legitimate. It utilises three different aspects of political legitimacy – input, output, and throughput legitimacy – to construct a 'legitimacy framework for the good use of evidence'. This framework identifies factors necessary to ensure the democratic legitimacy of evidence advisory systems, such as requiring evidence providing bodies to have a formal mandate (e.g. from government), ensuring that final policy decision-making authority lies with representatives of the public, and ensuring public transparency and deliberation in evidence-informed policy processes.

Finally, Chapter 8 brings together the multiple concepts addressed in the book to consider how to guide efforts to improve the use of evidence in policymaking. First, it discusses a range of institutional changes – both within and external to government – that can potentially help to address the politics of evidence and overcome bias. It then brings together the multiple normative discussions undertaken to construct a final framework of the good governance of evidence (see also an earlier discussion in Hawkins and Parkhurst (2015)). Rather than promoting a single model of evidence advice, the chapter argues that in order to ultimately improve the use of evidence for policymaking, it is essential to explicitly consider how to embed key principles of the good governance of evidence into those institutional arrangements shaping how evidence is utilised. Examples from various countries are provided, but the chapter ultimately promotes a process of 'guided evolution' that reflects a process of making incremental changes within a local context, informed by the principles within the good governance of evidence framework.

References

Adams, Michael. 2015. 'Crime and populism'. *Policy Options.* http://policyoptions.irpp.org/magazines/beautiful-data/adams, accessed 1 July 2016.

Banerjee, Neela, Lisa Song and David Hasemyer. 2015. 'Exxon – the road not taken'. http://insideclimatenews.org/content/Exxon-The-Road-Not-Taken, accessed 1 July 2016.

Barnes, Amy and Justin Parkhurst. 2014. 'Can global health policy be depoliticised? A critique of global calls for evidence-based policy'. In *Handbook of Global Health Policy*, edited by Gavin Yamey and Garrett Brown, pp. 157–173. Chichester: Wiley-Blackwell.

Barnes, Robert. 2016. 'Arguments in Supreme Court abortion case pitched to audience of one'. *Washington Post*, 29 February. https://www.washingtonpost.com/politics/courts_law/arguments-in-supreme-court-abortion-case-pitched-to-audience-of-one/2016/02/28/55d54998-dcbb-11e5-891a-4ed04f4213e8_story.html, accessed 1 July 2016.

Black, Nick. 2001. 'Evidence based policy: Proceed with care'. *British Medical Journal* 323: 275–279.

Brecht, Arnold. 1959. *Political Theory: The Foundations of Twentieth-Century Political Thought.* Princeton, NJ: Princeton University Press.

Chalmers, Iain. 2005. 'If evidence-informed policy works in practice, does it matter if it doesn't work in theory?' *Evidence & Policy: A Journal of Research, Debate and Practice* 1(2): 227–242. doi: 10.1332/1744264053730806.

Gilbert, Ruth, Georgia Salanti, Melissa Harden and Sarah See. 2005. 'Infant sleeping position and the sudden infant death syndrome: systematic review of observational studies and historical review of recommendations from 1940 to 2002'. *International Journal of Epidemiology* 34(4): 874–887.

Greenhalgh, Trisha and Jill Russell. 2009. 'Evidence-based policymaking: A critique'. *Perspectives in Biology and Medicine* 52(2): 304–318.

Hall, Shannon. 2015. 'Exxon knew about climate change almost 40 years ago'. *Scientific American.* http://www.scientificamerican.com/article/exxon-knew-about-climate-change-almost-40-years-ago, accessed 1 July 2016.

Hammersley, Martyn. 2005. 'Is the evidence-based practice movement doing more good than harm? Reflections on Iain Chalmers' case for research-based policy making and practice'. *Evidence & Policy: A Journal of Research, Debate and Practice* 1(1): 85–100.

——. 2013. *The Myth of Research-Based Policy and Practice*. London: Sage.

Hartnett, Stephen J. and Laura A. Stengrim. 2004. '"The whole operation of deception": Reconstructing President Bush's rhetoric of weapons of mass destruction'. *Cultural Studies↔Critical Methodologies* 4(2): 152–197.

Hawkins, Benjamin and Justin Parkhurst. 2015. 'The "good governance" of evidence in health policy'. *Evidence & Policy: A Journal of Research, Debate and Practice*. doi: 10. 1332/174426415X14430058455412.

Howick, Jeremy. 2011. *The Philosophy of Evidence-Based Medicine*. Oxford: Wiley-Blackwell.

Jamieson, Kathleen Hall. 2007. 'Justifying the war in Iraq: What the Bush administration's uses of evidence reveal'. *Rhetoric & Public Affairs* 10(2): 249–273.

Kumar, Sanjay. 2014. 'India's "yoga ministry" stirs doubts among scientists'. *Nature*. http://www.nature.com/news/india-s-yoga-ministry-stirs-doubts-among-scientists-1.16362, accessed 1 July 2016.

Lasswell, Harold Dwight. 1990 [1936]. *Politics: Who Gets What, When, How*. Gloucester, MA: Peter Smith Publishers.

Lewis, Jenny M. 2003. 'Evidence-based policy: A technocratic wish in a political world'. In *Evidence-Based Health Policy: Problems and Possibilities*, edited by Vivian Lin and Brendan Gibson, 250–259. Oxford: Oxford University Press.

Lin, Vivian. 2003. 'Competing rationalities: evidence-based health policy'. In *Evidence-Based Health Policy: Problems and Possibilities*, edited by Vivian Lin and Brendan Gibson, pp. 3–17. Oxford: Oxford University Press.

Lowndes, Vivian. 2010. 'The institutional approach'. In *Theory and Methods in Political Science*, edited by David Marsh and Gerry Stoker, 6–79. Basingstoke: Palgrave Macmillian.

Nutley, Sandra, Alison Powell and Huw Davies. 2013. *What Counts as Good Evidence?* London: Alliance for Useful Evidence.

Onthemedia. 2015. 'Exxon responds to InsideClimate News'. *WNYC Public Radio*. http://www.onthemedia.org/story/exxon-responds-insideclimate-news, accessed 1 July 2016.

Orritt, Rachel. 2014. 'Dog ownership has unknown risks but known health benefits: We need evidence-based policy'. *British Medical Journal* 349: 4081.

Parkhurst, Justin and Sudeepa Abeysinghe. 2016. 'What constitutes "good" evidence for public health and social policy-making? From hierarchies to appropriateness'. *Social Epistemology* 1–15. doi: 10.1080/02691728.2016.1172365.

Parsons, Wayne. 2002. 'From muddling through to muddling up: Evidence-based policy making and the modernisation of British government'. *Public Policy and Administration* 17(3): 43–60. doi: 10.1177/095207670201700304.

Partos, Rebecca. 2014. 'No immigrants, no evidence? The making of Conservative Party immigration policy'. *Political Insight*, 5: 12–15.

Peters, Guy. 2005. *Institutional Theory in Political Science*. London: Continuum.

Pfiffner, James P. 2004. 'Did President Bush mislead the country in his arguments for war with Iraq?' *Presidential Studies Quarterly* 34(1): 25–46.

Pielke, Roger A. 2002. 'Science policy: Policy, politics and perspective'. *Nature* 416(6879): 367–368.

Rittel, Horst W. J. and Melvin M. Webber. 1973. 'Dilemmas in a general theory of planning'. *Policy Sciences* 4(2): 155–169.

Rothstein, Bo. 1996. 'Political institutions: An overview'. In *A New Handbook of Political Science*, edited by Robert E. Goodin and Hans-Dieter Klingemann, 133–166. Oxford: Oxford University Press.

Russell, Jill, Trisha Greenhalgh, Emma Byrne and Janet McDonnell. 2008. 'Recognizing rhetoric in health care policy analysis'. *Journal of Health Services Research & Policy* 13(1): 40–46. doi: 10.1258/jhsrp.2007.006029.

Tenet, George J. 2003. 'Statement by George J. Tenet Director of Central Intelligence'. US Central Intelligence Agency. https://www.cia.gov/news-information/press-releases-statements/press-release-archive-2003/pr07112003.html, accessed 1 July 2016.

Weiss, Carol H. 1979. 'The many meanings of research utilization'. *Public Administration Review* 39(5): 426–431.

Wesselink, Anna, Hal Colebatch and Warren Pearce. 2014. 'Evidence and policy: Discourses, meanings and practices'. *Policy Sciences* 47(4): 339–344. doi: 10.1007/s11077-014-9209-2.

Wise, M. Norton. 2006. 'Thoughts on the politicization of science through commercialization'. *Social Research* 73(4): 1253–1272.

2 Evidence-based policymaking

An important first step and the need to take the next

The great potential for evidence to inform public policy

Chapter 1 explained that evidence matters. In many ways, of course, this is self-evident. For any decision and for any course of action, we will want information that tells us if we are achieving our goals, or to inform our selection of possible strategies to achieve our goals. Evidence is, by definition, what tells us these things (even if there may be debate over which goals to pursue in the first place). And so, in public policymaking, evidence can be useful for any number of decisions – from those as mundane as changing the timing of traffic lights to those as profound as a decision to go to war. And yet the rhetoric about the need for governments to do 'what works' under the banner of 'evidence-based policymaking' (EBP) has seen particularly widespread growth in recent years (Davies, Nutley and Smith 2000b; Nutley, Walter and Davies 2007).

However, this recognition of the usefulness of evidence is not exactly a new phenomenon. Some see the idea of EBP dating back at least to the 1950s, reflected in the work of American political scientist Harold Lasswell, who worked to identify the roles that research can play in addressing policy problems (Wesselink, Colebatch and Pearce 2014). Others trace a longer lineage. Hammersley, for example, claims that: 'The idea that evidence should inform political and social practice can be traced back at least as far as Machiavelli' (2013, p. 1), while Sutcliffe and Court explain that: 'As far back as ancient Greece, Aristotle put forward the notion that different kinds of knowledge should inform rulemaking' (2005, p. 1).

Yet, the modern engagement with the use of evidence to guide social policy grew significantly after the Second World War (Nutley, Walter and Davies 2007). Pawson and Tilley (1997) have described the growth of social policy evaluation and experimentation in the US in particular in this period. They reflect on large national programmes in fields such as early year education and crime prevention which were set up as experimental trials, as well as efforts to review evidence in order to draw lessons of 'what works' in these complex social policy realms. Berridge and Stanton (1999) similarly note the influence of social programme evaluation in the US in the 1960s, as well as other trends, such as the emphasis on planning and evaluation of international donor programmes seen in the 1970s, in shaping modern ideas of the role of evidence in policymaking.

Yet it was in the 1990s that many see the modern EBP movement taking shape. Some point to the explicit embrace of the concept by the UK Labour government of the time, which declared in its party manifesto of 1997 that 'what counts is what works' (Davies, Nutley and Smith 2000a; Parsons 2002). Others note the highly influential role of the establishment of the Cochrane Collaboration in 1993, which was developed to systematically organise and review evidence on medical and health interventions to provide a global repository for best practices in health care (Starr et al. 2009).

Indeed, the health sector is routinely cited as a key inspiration for many current calls for EBP today due to its development of the field of evidence-based medicine, which established how the choice of clinical interventions should be informed by rigorous research and a systematic review of effectiveness (cf. Berridge and Stanton 1999; Lin and Gibson 2003; Smith 2013; Wright, Parry and Mathers 2007). The US Coalition for Evidence-Based Policy (2015) reflects this desire to emulate the medical model when it explains:

> In the field of medicine, public policies based on scientifically rigorous evidence have produced extraordinary advances in health over the past 50 years. By contrast, in most areas of social policy – such as education, poverty reduction, and crime prevention – government programs often are implemented with little regard to evidence, costing billions of dollars yet failing to address critical social problems.

Young further notes that: 'The perceived success and value of [evidence-based medicine] stimulated an increasingly widespread interest in applying its fundamental principles to other fields and, indeed, to the realm of policy development in general' (2011, p. 20).

One of the fundamental principles embraced from the evidence-based medicine movement has been the use of experimental methods to evaluate interventions and measure effect, which has been seen to have revolutionised the medical field by serving to identify 'what works' in medical treatment. Everything from aspirin for migraines (cf. Boureau et al. 1994) to skin cancer treatments (cf. Robert et al. 2015) to the effectiveness of statins for heart disease (cf. Mills et al. 2011) have been tested through experimentation to judge their usefulness. Indeed, one of the simplest and cheapest medical interventions available – the use of oral rehydration solution (ORS) for diarrhoea – has been credited by the World Health Organization (WHO) with 'saving over 50 million children's lives' in the developing world (WHO 2009) after rigorous evaluation showed its usefulness in the 1970s (Munos, Walker and Black 2010).

And while research evidence can show the benefits of medical interventions, evidence can also stop the continued use of harmful treatments. In a historical reflection, Howick explains that until the mid-twentieth century, it was likely that most medical interventions 'were no better than placebo or positively harmful' (2011, p. 136). He argues that many medical procedures were only based on conceptual ideas of how something *might* work and, as such, may have led to more harm than good. He gives examples such as the advice on the sleeping position of babies (based on a flawed theory of the risk of choking) discussed in the previous chapter, as well as the historical use of bloodlettings (based on a flawed theory of the need to balance the 'blood humor') to illustrate the risk of basing interventions on hypothetical reasoning alone.

Champions of EBP have argued that just as medical interventions should be tested or evaluated using rigorous standards of evidence, so too should interventions in other social policy realms. Indeed, the perceived successes of the evidence-based medicine movement has made the health sector the envy of many other policy areas, with calls to embrace the 'medical model' now heard in areas such as education (Davies 1999; Slavin 2008), criminal justice (Sullivan, Hunter and Fisher 2013; Welsh and Farrington 2001), homelessness (Seibel 2011) and international development (International Initiative for Impact Evaluation 2010; Sutcliffe and Court 2005), amongst others. These ideas have also supported the establishment of formal governmental and non-governmental agencies that work to increase the use of evidence in policymaking. Examples include: the Coalition for Evidence-Based Policy, a US non-profit formed in 2001 'to increase government effectiveness through the use of rigorous evidence about what works' (Coalition for Evidence-Based Policy 2015),[1] Pakistan's Center for Economic Research (CERP), founded by international academic bodies in 2008 with the aim 'to promote the use of evidence-based decision-making among actors working towards social and economic development' (CERP 2013) or the UK's Alliance for Useful Evidence, a network that works for 'improving and extending the use of social research and evidence in the UK' (Alliance for Useful Evidence 2016) – and which lobbied to establish the UK's 'What Works Centres', a set of formal bodies created by the government to emulate the health sector model in providing guidelines and reviews of evidence of public service effectiveness in areas such as education, policing, ageing and local economic growth (What Works Network 2014).

However, it is not just any evidence that is promoted by such groups, as it has been noted that the term 'evidence' can refer to a great many things, ranging from tacit knowledge and personal experience to more systematic findings from organised professional inquiries and the outcomes of experiments (Nutley, Walter and Davies 2007; Weiss 1991). Instead, the EBP movement has particularly championed *scientific evidence* (arising from research) as the form best suited to inform policymaking. The US National Research Council (2012), for example, argues for the policy value of scientific evidence as follows:

> Science identifies problems – endangered species, obesity, unemployment, and vulnerability to natural disasters or bioterrorism or cyber attacks or bullying. It measures their magnitude and seriousness. Science offers solutions to problems, in some instances extending to policy design and implementation, from improved weapons systems to public health to school reform.

1 As of 2016, this agency has closed, with its core activities integrated into the Laura and John Arnold Foundation. See http://www.arnoldfoundation.org/initiative/evidence-based-policy-innovation.

> Science also predicts the likely outcomes of particular policy actions and then evaluates those outcomes, intended and unintended, wanted and unwanted. In these multiple ways science is of value to policy, *if used.*
>
> (2012, p. 7, emphasis in original)

Within these calls for increased use of scientific evidence, once-obscure terms such as 'randomised controlled trial', 'systematic review' and 'meta-analysis' have also become commonplace. Previously the reserve of clinical, epidemiological or evaluation science, many now argue that controlled experiments and evidence syntheses in these forms represent the 'gold standard' of knowledge upon which policies should be based, sitting at the top of 'hierarchies' of evidence that are, we are told, best suited to guide decision making (cf. Bigby 2009; Boaz, Ashby and Young 2002; Haynes, Goldacre and Torgerson 2012). Later discussion, particularly in Chapter 6, explores some of the challenges in applying such ideas to policymaking, but Box 2.1 provides a brief definition of some of these terms for readers who are unfamiliar with them.

Box 2.1 Selected evidence terminology

Randomised controlled trial (RCT) (also experimental trial, randomised trial or randomised clinical trial (in medicine)): these are experiments conducted in which an intervention is tested by randomly assigning some individuals, groups or regions to receive the intervention, and other areas not to do so (to be used as a 'control' group – either getting nothing or receiving another established intervention). In medical trials, this can mean giving some research subjects a new drug and others a placebo, while in social policy interventions, it might mean giving some regions a new service to compare with other areas that have not yet been provided with the service. The RCT design particularly helps to identify if an intervention has had an effect on outcomes, because the only difference between the (randomly assigned) treatment and control groups should be the intervention itself.

Systematic review: a form of literature review that aims to look at all existing work published about a topic and that attempts to follow particularly rigorous and transparent steps in doing so, such as identifying how materials will be found, which key words will be included and what types of literature will be included or excluded. Often these are applied to interventions to identify all possible data about a particular intervention in order to have the best information about its effectiveness (cf. Gough, Oliver and Thomas 2012; Petticrew and Roberts 2006).

Meta-analysis: related to systematic reviews, meta-analysis refers to the process of combining multiple studies of the same intervention in order to achieve greater certainty or clarity about its actual effect. Often this involves combining data from multiple randomised trials in order to essentially have a larger test population and larger body of evidence on which to judge intervention effect than would be possible from any single experimental trial alone.

The justification for the embrace of scientific evidence of this kind, of course, ultimately lies in the view that more rigorous and systematic uses of evidence will improve the effectiveness or efficiency of public policies, just as it has improved the effectiveness and efficiency of medical treatment. These forms of evidence are particularly placed at the top of so-called 'hierarchies' of evidence because they utilise rigorous methodology that is specifically designed to test or demonstrate evidence of effect (in the case of RCTs and meta-analyses in particular) and, as such, provide the best evidence of 'what works'. Greater use of evidence such as this is assumed to make it more likely to achieve programme goals, to obtain better outcomes for the population and to save valuable limited resources by selecting more effective or cost-effective solutions to social problems (Chalmers 2003; Davies, Nutley and Smith 2000b; Shepherd 2007).

What's wrong with 'what works'?

As noted above, given the success of modern medicine, calls and efforts to emulate the medical model now abound. For example, in 1997, the President of the UK Royal Statistical Society, Adrian Smith, reflected on the Cochrane Collaboration's successes in providing evidence to the medical field by stating:

> But what's so special about medicine? We are . . . confronted daily with controversy and debate across a whole spectrum of public policy issues. But, typically, we have no access to any form of systematic 'evidence base' – and therefore, no means of participating in the debate in a mature and informed manner. Obvious topical examples include education – what *does* work in the classroom? – and penal policy – what *is* effective in preventing reoffending?
>
> (Smith 1996, pp. 369–370, emphasis in original)

The idea of finding 'what works' is no doubt intuitively appealing, yet this quote appears to be unaware of the fact that the fields of education and crime prevention specifically did attempt to answer these questions with increasingly large experiments and reviews of data in the 1960s and 1970s, finding significant challenges to identifying any simple universal solutions (see Pawson and Tilley 1997: Chapter 1 of which provides a useful historical overview of these efforts). Furthermore, a political perspective highlights two key problems with the idea that we can simply look for evidence of 'what works' to guide public policy. The first, as discussed in the previous chapter, is that evidence alone tells us nothing about social desirability of that which is being measured, with the desired outcomes much less agreed upon for most social policy concerns than for clinical medicine. The second is that the language of doing 'what works' typically assumes and commonly implies a generalisability of effect that, while common in clinical medicine, is much less common in other policy relevant interventions.

What's wrong with what works (1): evidence of effect does not equate to social desirability

The political perspective used in this book starts from a recognition that policymaking is typically concerned with setting priorities and allocating scarce resources. In doing so, policy decisions typically involve choices between options containing multiple and competing sets of social values. From this perspective, when presented with evidence that something *works*, the natural response should not be to simply do it, but rather to ask: 'Works to do *what*, exactly?' In other words, presenting evidence that something is *effective* does not necessarily mean that it is *socially important*. And yet, in efforts to promote particular forms of evidence in order to prioritise policy options, there is a fundamental risk that the 'what works' language confuses certainty of effect with desirability of outcome.

Even within the health sector, a simple example illustrates this point. Below is a figure representing the results of a meta-analysis of a drug treatment. It shows that this particular drug was tested in no less than 16 randomised controlled trials, every single one of which found statistically significant positive effects compared to placebo (as indicated by the total point estimate and confidence-interval bars to the right of the vertical line in the fourth column).

This is overwhelmingly strong evidence of *what works*. It is the best-quality 'gold standard' evidence that many suggest should guide policymaking – not just one randomised trial, but 16 trials no less, every one of which showed significant positive results. So the provision of this drug should clearly be a high priority in health programmes and budgets . . . yes?

The answer, of course, is 'it depends'. It depends on what this drug is for and if it represents a social or health service priority. The pharmacologically aware reader will have noted that Figure 2.1 below presents data for the drug Sildenafil.

Comparison: 05 Sildenafil compared with placebo
Outcome: 01 Global Efficacy Question

Study	Experiment n/N	Control n/N	Risk difference (95% CI Random)	Weight %	Risk difference (95% CI Random)
101	202/310	22/74		6.6	0.354 (0.237 – 0.471)
102	209/293	53/194		8.0	0.440 (0.359 – 0.521)
103	101/136	23/141		7.5	0.580 (0.484 – 0.675)
104	74/131	13/127		7.3	0.463 (0.363 – 0.562)
106	262/338	27/108		7.5	0.525 (0.432 – 0.618)
351	10/12	2/12		2.4	0.667 (0.368 – 0.965)
353	186/242	35/91		6.8	0.384 (0.217 – 0.497)
355	36/44	10/44		4.9	0.591 (0.423 – 0.759)
356	81/99	28/106		6.8	0.554 (0.441 – 0.667)
357	11/21	2/21		3.1	0.429 (0.181 – 0.676)
358	18/27	2/27		4.0	0.593 (0.389 – 0.796)
359	42/52	7/39		5.1	0.628 (0.467 – 0.789)
361	128/167	6/47		6.7	0.639 (0.524 – 0.754)
363	117/142	29/121		7.3	0.584 (0.486 – 0.683)
364	276/359	27/114		7.7	0.532 (0.443 – 0.621)
367	142/175	21/174		8.2	0.691 (0.615 – 0.766)
Total (95% CI)	1895/2548	307/1440		100.0	0.537 (0.484 – 0.589)

$\chi^2 = 49.17$ (df = 15); $Z = 19.88$

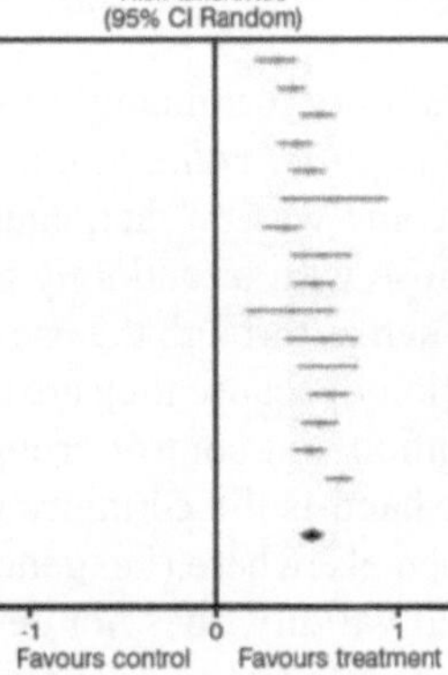

Figure 2.1 Results of a meta-analysis.

Source: Burls (2001), p. 1005, reproduced with permission.

This is sold under the brand name *Viagra* – a drug that has had a huge amount of money spent on it by corporate actors to prove through rigorous evaluation methods that it *works* for overcoming erectile dysfunction. The highest standard of effectiveness evidence exists for this drug. But if a government says 'what counts is what works' without asking 'to do what?', does this imply that what counts is fixing erectile dysfunction or that this goal should somehow have priority over the other important concerns the health budget might address, but for which there is weaker evidence? This may be an obvious case, but it is used to highlight the need to ensure that we do not sacrifice social priorities at the altar of methodological rigour.

What's wrong with what works (2): what works there *may not work* here

The second problem with the 'what works' language is that it typically implies certainty of causality or impact. The allure of the scientific method and rigorous testing of interventions through experimental trials is indeed intellectually seductive. Yet one of the most common errors made by those championing EBP is to assume that these evaluation methods tell us 'what works', with no further qualification mentioned.

The error in such statements is a failure to appropriately consider *generalisability*. There is a very big difference between finding that something works *when and where it was done* and the much larger (and often more important) question of whether it works *everywhere and always*. For policy relevance, evidence is needed that can provide certainty that an effect can be produced in the context where it is implemented. Sometimes this is the case, but often it is not. Cartwright and Hardie (2012) elaborate on this point further when they map out the differences between the questions of 'did it work somewhere?', 'will it work elsewhere?' and 'will it work for us?'. RCTs are designed to answer the first question, but policy decisions typically require evidence of the third question in particular.

This distinction is more technically referred to as the difference between the *internal validity* and *external validity* of a study. *Internal validity* is the certainty we have that an outcome was, in fact, caused by our intervention. Experimental trials, particularly those with a randomly assigned control group (and 'blinding' to the intervention, such as through the use of a placebo in drug trials), are good at ensuring internal validity because they are set up to ensure that the only difference between the intervention and control group was the intervention itself. *External validity* on the other hand is the certainty we have that the effect we saw in one location would happen elsewhere (i.e. generalisability).

Crucially, external validity does not derive from the method of experimentation; rather, it is other information we already know that lets us judge whether an experiment would work in the same way elsewhere. Consider experiments testing new medicines. The reason why we expect generalisability of results is because drugs work through biochemical and physiological mechanisms, and humans share their biochemistry and physiology. There will of course be some variance – with factors such as metabolism, co-infections or sex of the individual potentially influencing how (or how much) a medicine works. But we have a large evidence base about the similarities of human biochemistry, anatomy and physiology worldwide – an evidence base not necessarily derived from experiments, but rather from investigations of the human body and its functions. Medical drug trials are often assumed to be generalisable (externally valid) because we already know that many aspects of the human body function in the same way across a wide range of contexts.

However, at the opposite end of the spectrum, we can consider interventions where the effects are completely determined by local contextual elements that change according to place and time. In such cases, one can undertake experiments which are rigorously constructed, but which would not tell us anything outside the local context. An example might be in the area of fashion. Hypothetically, we could design an experimental trial to evaluate, for example, if changing the length of dresses from below or above the knee increases demand and hence sales. This experiment might be *internally* valid – we might have a good amount of certainty that any change in sales was due to our intervention. But would this experiment tell us 'what works' to increase dress sales? Would we expect the same results if we did it in different locations (say Sweden versus Saudi Arabia) or in the same place at different points in time (say the US in the 1950s versus the 1960s)? The external validity of an experiment on something as contextually driven as fashion would be very low, because the mechanism by which the intervention (altering dress length) causes the effect (sales) is determined by the context. This stands in contrast to biological interventions, whereby the biochemical mechanisms often remain the same (aspirin does, in fact, work through the same mechanism in Sweden as it does in Saudi Arabia and it worked in the same way in 1950s America as it did in 1960s America).

When the President of the Royal Statistical Society asked 'what is so special about medicine?', he apparently assumed the answer was 'nothing'. But the actual answer is 'quite a lot, really'. Medical interventions are based around biological and physiological mechanisms which are widely shared by humans. Many other interventions (like those to reduce crime or promote better educational outcomes) will function through socially embedded mechanisms that may not be common or that at least need some additional information to assume commonality across contexts. Medicine provides a great inspiration, but the human body is fundamentally different from a social environment.

The language of 'what works' therefore risks confusing internal and external validity. This, in turn, risks policies failing in practice if an internally valid result is assumed to be generalisable without sufficient supporting information. The failure to recognise that interventions may work in some places, but not in others can also undermine efforts to learn from the mixed results of multiple social policy evaluations. Pawson and Tilley (1997) describe this in a classic case of a 1974 systematic review of efforts to rehabilitate criminal offenders. In this review, Martinson (1974) found only 'isolated' instances of success. The paper was widely interpreted as finding 'nothing works' in the field, yet Pawson and Tilley note that *some* crime rehabilitation efforts work for *some* people in *some* situations. What is critical to know, in those cases, is how mechanisms of effect work in different contexts (what works for whom and where) rather than simply conducting more and more experiments in the hope of finding the one magic bullet that will work for all people in all cases (Pawson and Tilley 1997).

While evaluations remain key to measure if something has an effect, understanding mechanisms of effect matter too. Indeed, modern medicine relies heavily on understanding mechanisms of effect to know what to evaluate in the first place. For example, the most effective treatments for people living with HIV/AIDS are based on combinations of drugs that inhibit the virus in two or more different ways. Some drugs stop the virus attaching to cells, some stop the virus integrating into the cell, while some stop the virus replicating. Only by knowing mechanisms of how retroviruses (of which HIV is an example) propagate in the body could these different types of drugs be developed. So-called 'mechanistic reasoning' is incredibly important, yet evaluative evidence remains essential too. Only by rigorously testing the effectiveness of different combinations of antiretroviral drugs could we get to where we are today in HIV treatment, where a person receiving treatment for their HIV has a good chance of a long life expectancy (and likely to die of something other than AIDS) (Antiretroviral Therapy Cohort Collaboration 2010).

Bridging the gap between research and policy

Despite these problems with the idea of simply doing 'what works', the idea has been highly influential in supporting a wide range of efforts that aim to increase the use of evidence within policy. Such efforts are particularly based around the belief that there is a 'gap' between research and policy that must be bridged in order to achieve the great potential of scientific research evidence (Bennett and Jessani 2011; Cairney 2015; Van der Arend 2014). The former director of the World Health Organization, for instance, explained that: 'Scientifically excellent public health guidelines and other reliable information sit inert in journals and databases unless there is political commitment . . . to turning knowledge into action that will get results on the ground' (Lee 2003, p. 473). Similarly the United Nations Conference on Trade and Development (UNCTAD) has developed recommendations for 'bridging the gap between researchers and policy makers' (UNCTAD 2006, p. 1), explaining that: 'There tends to be a lack of communication between researchers and policy makers. Policy makers are not always informed about ongoing research and researchers often lack knowledge of the most pressing policy questions that they would need to make their research more relevant' (2006, p. 2).

However, this idea of a gap to be bridged dates back at least to the 1970s, when Caplan explained that:

> literature abounds with social scientists [*sic*] speculations about why information they produce has little impact on policy matters . . . the most prevalent theory found in this literature may be characterized as the 'Two-Communities' theory . . . Authors who hold this view attempt to explain non-utilization in terms of the relationship of the researcher and the research system to the policy maker and the policy-making system.
>
> (1979, p. 459)

This 'two communities' model has been the underlying concept behind a veritable cottage industry of work dedicated to some form of 'knowledge transfer', also referred to by linked terms such as knowledge mobilisation, knowledge translation, knowledge management, knowledge exchange and knowledge brokering (Davies, Powell and Nutley 2015; Shaxson et al. 2012). Common strategies under these headings particularly try to bring together researchers (or research results) and policy decision makers, including: 'research-push' efforts to improve the dissemination of evidence (such as by writing policy briefs and conducting systematic reviews); 'policy-pull' efforts to strengthen the capacity of policy makers to use research (e.g. by training decision makers on how to understand systematic reviews); or through 'bridging the gap' via linkage and exchange mechanisms that facilitate the transfer of information between sets of researchers and policy makers (Bennett and Jessani 2011; Lavis 2009; Start and Hovland 2004; SUPPORT Programme undated; UNCTAD 2006; World Health Organization undated).

There has even been at least one experimental evaluation of knowledge transfer efforts. Structured as a randomised controlled trial, Dobbins and colleagues (2009) tested whether different efforts at knowledge brokering were more or less effective with decision makers within Canadian public health departments. However, the study's findings were limited. They found no significant effect for their primary outcome (the extent to which research evidence was 'used' in a recent policy decision) and only a secondary effect from providing 'targeted, tailored messages' in broader programmatic decisions. The authors explain that the impact seen was mediated by the organisational culture of the department, concluding that there is a need for a greater understanding of organisational factors and of strategies that meet the needs of specific organisations.

Social science perspectives on evidence use and bridging the gap

The breadth and volume of work in this area has led to a number of attempts to review the literature to try to distil lessons of 'what works' for knowledge transfer, or to identify common 'barriers' or 'facilitators' to evidence use (cf. Contandriopoulos et al. 2010; Davies, Powell and Nutley 2015; Langer, Tripney and Gough 2016; Mitton et al. 2007; Oliver et al. 2014). Yet a number of academic authors have pointed to the conceptual challenges involved in the ways that evidence utilisation has been promoted or studied in this field. Oliver and colleagues, for instance, undertook a 'critical analysis of the literature', which concluded that: 'Much of the research in this area is theoretically naive, focusing primarily on the uptake of research evidence as opposed to evidence defined more broadly, and privileging academics' research priorities over those of policymakers' (2014, p. 1).

Similarly, Smith has synthesised a number of existing reviews to distil the most common recommendations to help improve knowledge use, such as ensuring that research is accessible, supporting relationships between researchers and decision makers, improving communication channels and providing incentives for evidence utilisation (pp. 20–21). But in reflecting on this body of work, she also notes that 'the most popular recommendations . . . focus on mechanisms for *increasing* the chances that particular research projects will be employed by policy makers. This is distinct from trying to *improve* the use of research in policy'. She further explains that 'an assumption which is implicit within a great deal of the scholarship on the relationship between research and policy [is] that the use of research is *a priori* a positive outcome' (2013, p. 23, emphases in original).

Indeed, one of the biggest challenges facing the knowledge transfer literature has ultimately been the fairly simplistic way in which evidence or research 'use' is discussed. Typically 'use' is discussed as a single binary variable – as if evidence can be 'used' or 'not used', 'taken up' or 'not taken up'. There is a further assumption that all actors would agree that research utilisation is a positive thing, as Smith explains in the above quote. However, as described in the previous chapter, critical authors note that there may in fact be many bodies of evidence relevant to a policy decision, with no simple agreement over which ones should be used or when. Social scientists have further explained that there can be many ways to conceptualise evidence use other than simply the direct uptake or implementation of findings from a particular research study. Much writing on this subject points to the work of Carol Weiss, who, in the 1970s, constructed a framework that classifies seven distinct models of 'research utilisation' for the social sciences, which are summarised below (Weiss 1979):

1 *Knowledge-driven* – research identifies problems, through basic science, to then solve using applied research (based on a natural science model).
2 *Problem-solving* – the most common model for 'research utilisation' thinking, which 'involves the direct application of the results of a specific social science study to a pending decision' (Weiss 1979, p. 427).
3 *Interactive* – a back-and-forth process of learning between policy makers and multiple sources of information, including research.
4 *Political* – research used as 'ammunition' for pre-decided policy positions.
5 *Tactical* – research undertaken to deflect criticism or to show that 'something' is being done, even if the findings are irrelevant.
6 *Enlightenment* – an indirect way through which social science research influences thinking more broadly or generally, including working to identify problems or convert them into 'non-problems'.
7 Part of the *social intellectual enterprise* – social science research as an intellectual pursuit of society, responding to the 'fads and fancies' of the time.

In 2007 Nutley et al. further produced a comprehensive volume exploring the many ways through which research informs public services. They include Weiss' seven meanings of research use, but similarly describe a number of other typologies that have been developed over the years. The authors note that a common distinction made in such typologies is between *instrumental* use – seeing research directly influence policy and practice – and *conceptual* use, which captures 'the complex and often indirect ways in which research can have an impact on the knowledge, understanding, and attitudes of policy makers and practitioners' (2007, p. 36). Nutley et al. explain that it is policy makers in particular who use research in strategic and technical ways, noting that: 'Policy makers say that while research is often interesting and helpful . . . it most often "informs" policy, rather than providing a clear steer for action' (2007, p. 37).

Despite this fairly extensive body of work mapping out the multiple ways in which research can be utilised in policy processes, the EBP literature still overwhelmingly reflects the idea that evidence use is a technical problem-solving exercise (Greenhalgh and Russell 2009). However, this focus on problem solving shows its limitations quite quickly when considering how few policy decisions actually fit this model. Cairney, for example, refers to the EBP approach as capturing an idea of 'comprehensive rationality' of an 'optimal' policy process – a situation which rests on a large number of 'rather unrealistic assumptions about who is involved, what they represent, and the best way to make policy' (2015, p. 15). Similarly, Weiss herself explains that:

> It probably takes an extraordinary concatenation of circumstances for research to influence policy decisions directly: a well defined decision situation, a set of policy actors who have responsibility and jurisdiction for making the decision, an issue whose resolution depends at least to some extent on information, identification of the requisite informational need, research that provides the information in terms that match the circumstances within which choices will be made, research findings that are clear-cut, unambiguous, firmly supported, and powerful, that reach decision-makers at the time they are wrestling with the issues, that are comprehensible and understood, and that do not run counter to strong political interests. Because [the] chances are small that all these conditions will fall into line around any one issue, the problem-solving model of research use probably describes a relatively small number of cases.
>
> (1979, p. 428)

Yet, somehow, this 'relatively small number of cases' has become the template for the vast majority of work aiming to improve how evidence informs policy.

Applying theories of the policy process

To move beyond the simple problem-solving model, some academics have looked deeper into the field of policy studies to bring what Cairney (2015) calls the 'science of policymaking' to the question of evidence use (see also Lin and Gibson 2003; Smith 2013). So, for example, in his recent book, Cairney employs a broad body of policy studies theories and concepts in order to help explain evidence use within two specific policy areas – environmental policy and health and advocacy. Theories and approaches he draws on include the following:

- John Kingdon's (1995) 'multiple streams' model of policy change and 'punctuated equilibrium' theory, which emphasises the time dimension in evidence use and recognises that evidence may influence policy at key moments or alternatively only after long periods of time.
- 'Social construction theory' and the 'narrative policy framework', which emphasise the importance of the framing of a policy issue in shaping how evidence is used or what evidence is seen to be relevant.
- The 'advocacy coalitions framework', which highlights how evidence can be utilised within a process of policy change that reflects competition between rival groups and where policy stakeholders' belief systems work to shape the relevance of evidence.
- Studies of 'policy transfer, diffusion and learning', which highlight the importance of local political context and the generalisability of efforts to replicate or emulate policy activities in other settings.
- 'Complexity theory', which particularly warns against assumptions of predictability across decision-making systems (including in the use of evidence). A number of features of complex systems that are seen to be relevant to shaping how evidence is used include the presence of positive and negative feedback processes, the importance of initial conditions and path dependency, and emergent outcomes based on multiple interactions of actors within the system.

Smith follows a similar approach, drawing on many of these same policy theories to explore how research influences two particular public health case studies: those of tobacco control and health inequalities. In her review of policy concepts, she places particular emphasis on ideational theories that focus on how policy paradigms, policy frames and policy solutions all end up being constructed with reference to evidence. She concludes that, for her cases, 'it makes more sense to study the political influence of *ideas* than *evidence*' (2013, p. 108, emphasis in original).

A final example of authors applying policy studies theories to study evidence use can be seen in a slightly earlier volume edited by Lin and Gibson (2003), which explores evidence use in health policy. In one chapter, for instance, Gibson draws on a range of political theories, including David Dery's idea of 'organisational epistemology' and Michel Foucault's ideas of 'governmentality', to critique the 'two communities' model of evidence use as failing to capture the nature of health policy change (Gibson 2003). In the same volume, Lewis utilises Kingdon's 'policy streams' model to describe the process of policy change, while focusing on argumentation and framing theories to emphasise the importance of these discursive practices in shaping evidence use (Lewis 2003).

It is, perhaps, remarkable to see just how large a number of theories are drawn upon to help us understand evidence use within policy decisions. Yet one explanation for this is due to the fundamentally complex and multifaceted nature of the policy process into which evidence is expected to fit. Policy change involves individuals pursuing their interests, but it also involves networks working together, as well as the discursive construction of those interests in the first place. Policymaking can be driven by ideas, but it can also be shaped or constrained by institutional arrangements. All of these features can therefore be important with regard to evidence utilisation, and different theories and models may be applied to consider each of them. John (1998) provides a useful overview of the different approaches of the field of policy studies, noting that, in addition to well-established bodies of theories focusing on interests, ideas, institutions and networks, there are also cross-cutting theories of the policy process that have been developed to help explain policy change. However, he notes that no single one of these can explain all aspects of policymaking; rather, as Cairney (2007) has expressed, they provide 'multiple lenses' by which to understand different features of the policy process.

Policy theories can therefore be immensely useful in understanding evidence use from the perspective of describing policy change. Yet while this book shares conceptual origins with some of these other recent works, the focus here is different in one key respect. Other authors have particularly drawn on policy studies theories to conduct analyses of the utilisation of evidence in specific case studies of policy change. In contrast, this book began from a concern over the political origins of the two forms of bias detailed in Chapter 1: *technical bias*, in which evidence is misused or manipulated for political reasons; and *issue bias*, in which appeals to evidence serve to obscure key social values or impose political priority in unrepresentative ways. Therefore, our focus here is not so much on empirical analysis of a case study of policy change, but rather on addressing the question of how to improve the use of evidence in policy more generally.

Taking the next steps to improve the use of evidence

However, improving the use of evidence is a decidedly normative goal. For the EBP field, a principal impetus lies in the belief that greater fidelity to scientific good practice, reduced manipulation or misuse of evidence and increased application of science will lead to improved social policy outcomes – be it in terms of lives saved, better educational achievement or reduced criminal behaviour. Yet, the discussion above raises fundamental questions about what an 'improved' use of evidence actually looks like, given the political nature of policymaking. As noted by Smith (2013), the EBP movement has championed one particular idea which assumes that *more* use is *better* use, especially if that evidence comes from the top of particular hierarchies. However, previous discussions identified this approach as problematic due to the way in which it can, in the name of promoting technical effectiveness, work to depoliticise policy debates that need to reflect the multiple competing social values of a population. Both sides of this issue are concerned with the politics of evidence, but they reflect two distinct and equally important normative principles: fidelity to science on the one hand and democratic representation on the other.

The approach of this book is to consider how to improve the use of evidence in reference to both these principles, but with a more explicit recognition of the nature of politics that has been missing from much previous work promoting evidence use. The book is therefore normatively oriented and conceptually informed, but also aims to be decidedly pragmatic. It does not reject the EBP movement in its entirety, even if it is critical of the way in which EBP has at times been promoted. Some approaches to evidence use may appear oversimplified or politically naïve, but this does not mandate a complete rejection of the ultimate goal of improving the way in which evidence is used to achieve policy goals. Instead, in order to address the politics of evidence – in all its forms – we need to move beyond past efforts focusing solely on knowledge transfer, recognising that social goals can be contested, and understanding how the pursuit of our values may manifest in biased uses of evidence. So while the EBP movement is recognised to have taken an important first step in thinking about the need to improve evidence use, it is argued here that it is time to take the next steps as follows:

The need to address the political sources of technical and issue bias

Given the EBP community's concern with the political misuse of evidence, one of the most important limitations of current knowledge transfer efforts is their inability to actually address the political origins of many forms of evidentiary bias. When evidence is misused in *technically biased* ways, EBP champions decry politics as a corrupting influence and argue that if only more evidence were used appropriately, this could be avoided. Yet the strategy of providing more evidence to policy actors, training decision makers or linking the 'two worlds' cannot address political bias when such efforts are based upon a problem-solving model of evidence utilisation that assumes a universal desire to use evidence accurately. Similarly, knowledge transfer strategies are largely unable to address the concept of *issue bias* that can arise when promotion of evidence skews agendas to those issues which are measured rather than those which are important to affected populations. Indeed, from a political perspective, it is not surprising that the Canadian randomised trial of knowledge-brokering techniques was unable to definitively identify a knowledge transfer strategy as most effective (Dobbins et al. 2009). Different policy decisions will require different forms of evidence at different times. Nothing can be said to simply 'work' to inform policy when the policy involves more than a simple technical exercise.

When outcomes are not pre-agreed, the technical solutions promoted by knowledge transfer efforts further risk not only ignoring, but also potentially *imposing* issue bias if they promote a hierarchy of evidence that only speaks to a limited selection of relevant policy concerns. Training decision makers about experimental trials, for example, and emphasising that such trials are the 'best' way to make policy decisions, can implicitly shift political priorities towards those things on which experiments have already been done or which are conducive to experimentation (things like *Viagra*). The need to more directly address the political sources of both technical bias and issue bias is critical and the second part of this book (Chapters 3–5) explores these issues in greater depth.

The need to understand 'good evidence for policy': beyond hierarchies

As already noted, one of the most fundamental conceptual holdovers from the field of medicine within the EBP movement has been the primacy given to particular forms of evidence, in particular the randomised trial (Haynes, Goldacre and Torgerson 2012; Shepherd 2007) and the embrace of evidence hierarchies. Indeed, Annex 1 of Nutley, Powell and Davies (2013) contains a list of 15 examples of hierarchies or ranking systems to judge evidence that are applied in a range of social policy spheres, including health care, education, criminal justice and youth services. The authors note that these hierarchies are designed to rank evidence based on the study design, but their application has been shown to raise a number of challenges in terms of how such hierarchies may ignore other important evidence sources, may fail to recognise the need for local applicability or may provide an insufficient basis for policy decisions.

The main issue is not that RCTs and hierarchies are inherently flawed, but rather that they are being incorrectly applied in many cases if they are used to prioritise policy choices. As such, appeals to hierarchies can impose issue bias if they result in prioritising those social concerns conducive to experimentation or where stakeholders have already conducted experiments (Barnes and Parkhurst 2014). Over-reliance on hierarchies can also obscure the importance of external validity, often failing to explicitly address questions of the applicability of findings across contexts. While some authors have noted the limitations of hierarchies of evidence in terms of policy usefulness (cf. Cartwright and Hardie 2012; Parkhurst and Abeysinghe 2016; Petticrew and Roberts 2003), these ideas have yet to be taken up widely in the EBP movement. There still needs to be critical reflection upon what hierarchies can be used for and what 'good evidence for policy' would have to look like if single hierarchies do not meet the needs for evidence use within policy decisions. Chapter 6 in particular explores this question by defining good evidence for policy based on a concept of policy 'appropriateness'. Rather than promoting one hierarchy relevant to a single consideration, appropriate evidence is defined as that collection of evidence which addresses the multiple relevant political concerns, which is created to best serve policy needs and which is applicable in the local context.

The need to consider the 'good use of evidence' with respect to political legitimacy

Another relevant challenge to the EBP movement in achieving its ultimate goal of having scientific evidence improve social outcomes is to recognise the importance of the legitimacy of the decision-making processes utilising evidence. Too often the EBP literature seems to assume that evidence use is a universally embraced good thing – that using more evidence, or more of a particular form of evidence, will naturally be embraced by all the parties involved. Yet from a policy studies perspective, the process by which public policy decisions are made and social outcomes are achieved must be accepted as legitimate by the population.

Greenhalgh and Russell explain that: 'The very expression "evidence-based policy making" suggests that there are technical solutions to what are essentially political problems – an assumption that, some have argued, devalues democratic debate' (2006, p. 37). This importance placed on democratic debate reflects an understanding that the legitimacy of the decision-making process itself can be important to ensure that final policy decisions are respected. Yet in the EBP world, almost no attention has been paid to the legitimacy of the process through which evidence is applied. The focus has been on research 'use' or 'uptake', with competing political or cultural considerations simply classified as 'barriers' to be overcome, or with 'resistance' to evidence explained as being due to lack of understanding of the science by the potential beneficiaries (Oliver et al. 2014; Oliver, Lorenc and Innvaer 2014; Parkhurst, Chilongozi and Hutchinson 2015).

This is particularly striking given that some advocates of EBP have argued that evidence use can work to improve *governance*. The Organisation for Economic Co-operation and Development (OECD), for instance, has stated that 'good-governance practice suggests that policy should be based on sound evidence derived from rigorous analysis of the available facts on the issue that the policy is supposed to address' (OECD 2013, p. 149). Duckett further notes that the emergence of evidence-based health policy was in part driven by 'the development of greater accountability in public sector management' (2003, p. xv), and Davies, Nutley and Smith (2000b) argue that pressure to embrace EBP can come from an increasingly well-informed public. Indeed, the science author Ben Goldacre has gone so far as to state: 'I think we can improve democracy by improving the way we use data' (*BBC Newsnight* 2015).

But simply using evidence does not necessarily make a decision democratically legitimate. When pieces of technically valid evidence are used by corrupt authoritarian leaders, this illustrates the point. Indeed, the famous saying that Italian fascist leader Benito Mussolini 'made the trains run on time' serves as a warning that technical effectiveness is not a substitute for democratic governance. The distinction is important and Chapter 7 reflects on what principles of political legitimacy applied to evidence use might look like from the perspective of democratic representation in particular.

The need to build institutions to improve evidence use

Finally, if the EBP movement is ultimately driven by a concern to use evidence to help achieve social policy goals, there will be an obvious need to ensure that improvements will have lasting effects over time. However, the vast majority of work attempting to promote evidence use through knowledge transfer mechanisms has consisted of strategies targeting individuals: training researchers in how to provide information in more 'usable' ways; training decision makers in how to find or understand research evidence; or building links between them in a particular place and time (Mitton et al. 2007; Nutley, Walter and Bland 2002; Ward, House and Hamer 2009). The broader literature in this field similarly often focuses on the linking roles that individuals can play – serving as information intermediaries, knowledge providers, knowledge brokers and the like – although it should be noted that there are some authors who look further to identify how organisations might serve knowledge brokering-roles as well (Lavis et al. 2003; Lomas 2007; Shaxson et al. 2012).

A heavy focus on individuals as the driving force to improve the use of evidence in policymaking raises two particular issues. The first has to do with the roles of researchers, who are under increasing pressure to ensure that the research evidence they produce is 'used' or 'taken up'. This risks encouraging researchers to have political influence, a role that they are neither trained to do nor one that many feel they have the mandate to take on. The second problem is that such efforts can have a limited duration of impact, given that both researchers and decision makers will naturally change over time or move on from existing positions.

An alternative approach is to focus on the *institutionalisation* of changes that serve to improve evidence use, which Nutley and colleagues (2002) have similarly argued can help move beyond the individualistic focus of past strategies to link evidence and policy. Indeed, the medical model is seen as being so widely successful not only because it trained individual clinicians in evidence-based medicine, but also because it established broader institutional arrangements which could promote evidence use of a particular kind, and it further established norms and expectations of evidence use that have become commonplace in medical practice today.

This is not to say that there are no instances of institutional approaches to improving evidence use outside the health sector. The Cochrane Collaboration's success in establishing a repository for evidence of medical effectiveness has been emulated in the formation of the Campbell Collaboration, which attempts to similarly build an evidence base on the effectiveness of interventions in other social policy fields (Petrosino et al. 2001). There have also been examples of 'toolkits' designed to serve as good practice guidelines for either researchers or policymakers (cf. Bennett and Jessani 2011; Oxman et al. 2009; Start and Hovland 2004), and there are authors who have explored the role of knowledge brokering structures such as think tanks or knowledge translation platforms (Lavis et al. 2008, 2013; (Mendizabal and Sample 2009) that exist outside of any individual knowledge-brokering efforts. These represent important examples, but a much more explicit consideration of institutions will be needed by the EBP community to improve the use of evidence in social policymaking more broadly. Such an approach requires shifting thinking to consider *systems of evidence advice* rather than just targeting individuals as knowledge brokers.

Evidence-advisory *systems* can therefore broadly be conceptualised as the collection of structural bodies, rules and norms of practice which serve to govern the ways in which evidence informs policy decisions. These systems can be designed to reduce particular forms of evidentiary bias, yet their functioning can also serve to embed key principles and best practices of evidence use more broadly as well. Chapter 8 concludes this book by reflecting on many of the institutional shapes and forms that such efforts can take, noting that no single system or body will fit in all countries. Instead it reflects on the need to take steps to incrementally improve evidence advisory systems within different country institutional contexts and in line with explicit consideration of the normative principles of the good governance of evidence developed throughout the book.

Conclusion

This chapter has reflected on how the embrace of EBP, growing from its origins in evidence-based medicine, has been an important first step in thinking about how to improve evidence use, but we are now at a point where it is necessary to move forward. The EBP movement has embraced the social potential of increased application of science, but has risked doing so with insufficient understanding of the nature of the policy process and the normative concerns inherent to political decision making.

This book takes the EBP discussion forward by considering how to improve the use of evidence in ways that serve to promote the key normative principles of both scientific fidelity and democratic representation. Achieving this will require several steps along the way. First, there is a need to understand and explore the political origins of both technical bias and issue bias within policymaking settings. Once this is understood, we can then reflect more deeply about how to judge 'good evidence' within policymaking and the 'good use of evidence' from a perspective of the decision-making process. It is then necessary to reflect on how to achieve sustainable changes to improve evidence use over time in line with these multiple principles. This book argues that such an approach requires critically thinking about how to go about establishing evidence advisory systems that can ensure that rigorous, systematic and valid pieces of evidence are utilised within decision-making processes that remain representative of and accountable to local populations. This serves as an alternative way of thinking about how to improve evidence use, directly addressing the politics of evidence and moving from evidence-based policy towards the good governance of evidence.

References

Alliance for Useful Evidence. 2016. 'About us'. http://www.alliance4usefulevidence.org/about-us/aboutus, accessed 2 July 2016.

Antiretroviral Therapy Cohort Collaboration. 2010. 'Causes of death in HIV-1-infected patients treated with antiretroviral therapy, 1996–2006: Collaborative analysis of 13 HIV cohort studies'. *Clinical Infectious Diseases* 50(10): 1387–1396. doi: 10.1086/652283.

Barnes, Amy and Justin Parkhurst. 2014. 'Can global health policy be depoliticised? A critique of global calls for evidence-based policy'. In *Handbook of Global Health Policy*, edited by Gavin Yamey and Garrett Brown, pp. 157–173. Chichester: Wiley-Blackwell.

BBC Newsnight. 2015. 'Democracy Rewired', 4 February. http://www.bbc.co.uk/programmes/b006mk25/episodes/guide, accessed 1 July 2016.

Bennett, Gavin and Nasreen Jessani. 2011. *The Knowledge Translation Toolkit: Bridging the Know-Do gap: A Resource for Researchers*. New Delhi: Sage.

Berridge, V. and J. Stanton. 1999. 'Science and policy: Historical insights'. *Social Science & Medicine* 49(9): 1133–1138.

Bigby, Michael. 2009. 'The hierarchy of evidence'. *Evidence-Based Dermatology* 2: 34–37.

Boaz, Annette, Deborah Ashby and Ken Young. 2002. *Systematic Reviews: What Have They Got to Offer Evidence-Based Policy and Practice?* London: ESRC UK Centre for Evidence Based Policy and Practice.

Boureau, F., J.M. Joubert, V. Lasserre, B. Prum and G. Delecoeuillerie. 1994. 'Double-blind comparison of an acetaminophen 400 mg-codeine 25 mg combination versus aspirin 1000 mg and placebo in acute migraine attack'. *Cephalalgia* 14(2): 156–161.

Burls, Amanda, Lisa Gold and Wendy Clark. 2001. 'Systematic review of randomised controlled trials of sildenafil (Viagra) in the treatment of male erectile dysfunction'. *British Journal of General Practice* 51(473): 1004–1012.

Cairney, Paul. 2007. 'A "multiple lenses" approach to policy change: The case of tobacco policy in the UK'. *British Politics* 2: 45–68.

——. 2015. *The Politics of Evidence-Based Policymaking*. London: Palgrave Macmillan.

Caplan, Nathan. 1979. 'The two-communities theory and knowledge utilization'. *American Behavioral Scientist* 22(3): 459–470. doi: 10.1177/000276427902200308.

Cartwright, N. and J. Hardie. 2012. *Evidence-Based Policy: A Practical Guide to Doing it Better*. Oxford: Oxford University Press.

CERP. 2013. 'About CERP'. http://cerp.org.pk/aboutcerp, accessed 1 July 2016.

Chalmers, Iain. 2003. 'Trying to do more good than harm in policy and practice: The role of rigorous, transparent, up-to-date evaluations'. *Annals of the American Academy of Political and Social Science* 589(1): 22–40.

Coalition for Evidence-Based Policy. 2015. 'Our Mission'. http://coalition4evidence.org.

Contandriopoulos, Damien, Marc Lemire, Jean-Louis Denis and Émile Tremblay. 2010. 'Knowledge exchange processes in organizations and policy arenas: A narrative systematic review of the literature'. *Milbank Quarterly* 88(4): 444–483. doi: 10.1111/j.1468-0009.2010.00608.x.

Davies, Huw, Sandra Nutley and Peter Smith. 2000a. 'Introducing evidence-based policy and practice in public services'. In *What Works? Evidence-Based Policy and Practice in Public Services*, edited by Huw Davies, Sandra Nutley and Peter Smith, pp. 1–12. Bristol: Polity Press.

Davies, Huw, Sandra Nutley and Peter Smith. 2000b. *What Works? Evidence-Based Policy and Practice in Public Services*. Bristol: Polity Press.

Davies, Huw, Alison Powell and Sandra Nutley. 2015. 'Mobilising knowledge to improve UK health care: Learning from other countries and other sectors – a multimethod mapping study'. *Health Services Delivery Research* 3(27): 1–220.

Davies, Philip. 1999. 'What is evidence-based education?' *British Journal of Educational Studies* 47(2): 108–121.

Dobbins, Maureen, Steven Hanna, Donna Ciliska, Steve Manske, Roy Cameron, Shawna Mercer, Linda O'Mara, Kara DeCorby and Paula Robeson. 2009. 'A randomized controlled trial evaluating the impact of knowledge translation and exchange strategies'. *Implementation Science* 4(1): 61–77.

Duckett, Stephen. 2003. 'Foreword'. In *Evidence-Based Health Policy: Problems and Possibilities*, edited by Vivian Lin and Brendan Gibson, pp. xv–xvi. Oxford: Oxford University Press.

Gibson, Brendan. 2003. 'Beyond "two communities"'. In *Evidence-Based Health Policy: Problems and Possibilities*, edited by Vivian Lin and Brendan Gibson, pp. 18–30. Oxford: Oxford University Press.

Gough, David, Sandy Oliver and James Thomas. 2012. *An Introduction to Systematic Reviews*. London: Sage.

Greenhalgh, Trisha and Jill Russell. 2006. 'Reframing evidence synthesis as rhetorical action in the policy making drama'. *Healthcare Policy* 1(2): 34–42.

——. 2009. 'Evidence-based policymaking: A critique'. *Perspectives in Biology and Medicine* 52(2): 304–318.

Hammersley, Martyn. 2013. *The Myth of Research-Based Policy and Practice*. London: Sage.

Haynes, Laura, Ben Goldacre and David Torgerson. 2012. *Test, Learn, Adapt: Developing Public Policy with Randomised Controlled Trials*. London: Cabinet Office-Behavioural Insights Team.

Howick, Jeremy. 2011. *The Philosophy of Evidence-Based Medicine*. Oxford: Wiley-Blackwell.

International Initiative for Impact Evaluation. 2010. *Providing Evidence to Inform Policy: Annual Report 2010*. London: International Initiatuve for Impact Evaluation.

John, Peter. 1998. *Analysing Public Policy*. London: Continuum.

Kingdon, John W. 1995. *Agendas, Alternatives and Public Policies*. New York: Longman.

Langer, Laurenz, Janice Tripney and David Gough. 2016. *The Science of Using Science: Researching the Use of Research Evidence in Decision-Making*. London: EPPI-Centre, Social Science Research Unit, UCL Institution of Education, University College London.

Lavis, John N. 2009. 'How can we support the use of systematic reviews in policymaking?' *PLoS Medicine* 6(11): e1000141.

Lavis, John, Ray Moynihan, Andrew Oxman and Elizabeth Paulsen. 2008. 'Evidence-informed health policy 4: Case descriptions of organizations that support the use of research evidence'. *Implementation Science* 3(1): 56–65

Lavis, John N., Govin Permanand, Cristina Catallo and BRIDGE Study Team. 2013. *How Can Knowledge Brokering Be Advanced in a Country's Health System?* Copenhagen: World Health Organization.

Lavis, John N., Dave Robertson, Jennifer M. Woodside, Christopher B. McLeod and Julia Abelson. 2003. 'How can research organizations more effectively transfer research knowledge to decision makers?' *Milbank Quarterly* 81(2): 221–248. doi: 10.1111/1468-0009.t01-1-00052.

Lee, Jong-Wook. 2003. 'Science and the health of the poor'. *Bulletin of the World Health Organization* 81(7): 473.

Lewis, Jenny M. 2003. 'Evidence-based policy: A technocratic wish in a political world'. In *Evidence-Based Health Policy: Problems and Possibilities*, edited by Vivian Lin and Brendan Gibson, pp. 250–259. Oxford: Oxford University Press.

Lin, Vivian and Brendan Gibson, eds. 2003. *Evidence-Based Health Policy: Problems and Possibilities*. Oxford: Oxford University Press.

Lomas, Jonathan. 2007. 'The in-between world of knowledge brokering'. *British Medical Journal* 334: 129–132.

Martinson, Robert. 1974. 'What works? Questions and answers about prison reform'. *The Public Interest* 35(2): 22–54.

Mendizabal, Enrique and Kristen Sample. 2009. *Thinking Politics: Think Tanks and Political Parties in Latin America*. London: Overseas Development Institute.

Mills, E.J., P. Wu, G. Chong, I. Ghement, S. Singh, E.A. Akl, O. Eyawo, G. Guyatt, O. Berwanger and M. Briel. 2011. 'Efficacy and safety of statin treatment for cardiovascular disease: A network meta-analysis of 170 255 patients from 76 randomized trials'. *QJM*, 104: 109–124.

Mitton, Craig, Carol Adair, Emily McKenzie, Scott Patten and Brenda Waye Perry. 2007. 'Knowledge transfer and exchange: Review and synthesis of the literature'. *Milbank Quarterly* 85(4): 729–768. doi: 10.1111/j.1468-0009.2007.00506.x.

Munos, Melinda, Christa Fischer Walker and Robert Black. 2010. 'The effect of oral rehydration solution and recommended home fluids on diarrhoea mortality'. *International Journal of Epidemiology* 39(1): i75–i87. doi: 10.1093/ije/dyq025.

National Research Council. 2012. *Using Science as Evidence in Public Policy*. Edited by Kenneth Prewitt, Thomas A. Schwandt and Miron L. Straf. Washington DC: National Academies Press.

Nutley, Sandra, Alison Powell and Huw Davies. 2013. *What Counts as Good Evidence?* London: Alliance for Useful Evidence.

Nutley, Sandra, Isabel Walter and Nick Bland. 2002. 'The institutional arrangements for connecting evidence and policy: The case of drug misuse'. *Public Policy and Administration* 17(3): 76–94.

Nutley, Sandra, Isabel Walter and Huw Davies. 2007. *Using Evidence: How Research Can Inform Public Services*. Bristol: Policy Press.

OECD. 2013. 'Colombia: Implementing good governance'. In *OECD Public Governance Reviews*. Paris: OECD.

Oliver, Kathryn, Simon Innvar, Theo Lorenc, Jenny Woodman and James Thomas. 2014. 'A systematic review of barriers to and facilitators of the use of evidence by policymakers'. *BMC Health Services Research* 14(1): 2. doi: 10.1186/1472-6963-14-2.

Oliver, Kathryn, Theo Lorenc and Simon Innvaer. 2014. 'New directions in evidence-based policy research: A critical analysis of the literature'. *Health Research Policy and Systems* 12(1): 34. doi: 10.1186/1478-4505-12-34.

Oxman, Andrew, John Lavis, Simon Lewin and Atle Fretheim. 2009. 'SUPPORT Tools for evidence-informed health Policymaking (STP) 1: What is evidence-informed policymaking?' *Health Research Policy and Systems* 7 (1): S1.

Parkhurst, Justin, David Chilongozi and Eleanor Hutchinson. 2015. 'Doubt, defiance and identity: Understanding resistance to male circumcision for HIV prevention in Malawi'. *Social Science & Medicine* 135: 15–22.

Parkhurst, Justin and Sudeepa Abeysinghe. 2016. 'What constitutes "good" evidence for public health and social policy-making? From hierarchies to appropriateness'. *Social Epistemology* 1–15. doi: 10.1080/02691728.2016.1172365.

Parsons, Wayne. 2002. 'From muddling through to muddling up: Evidence-based policy making and the modernisation of British government'. *Public Policy and Administration* 17(3): 43–60. doi: 10.1177/095207670201700304.

Pawson, Ray and Nick Tilley. 1997. *Realistic Evaluation*. London: Sage.

Petrosino, Anthony, Robert Boruch, Haluk Soydan, Lorna Duggan and Julio Sanchez-Meca. 2001. 'Meeting the challenges of evidence-based policy: The Campbell Collaboration'. *Annals of the American Academy of Political and Social Science* 578(1): 14–34. doi: 10.1177/000271620157800102.

Petticrew, Mark and Helen Roberts. 2003. 'Evidence, hierarchies and typologies: Horses for courses'. *Journal of Epidemiology and Community Health* 57(7): 527–529.

——. 2006. *Systematic Reviews in the Social Sciences: A Practical Guide*. Malden, MA: Blackwell Publishing.

Robert, Caroline, Boguslawa Karaszewska, Jacob Schachter, Piotr Rutkowski, Andrzej Mackiewicz, Daniil Stroiakovski, Michael Lichinitser, Reinhard Dummer, Florent Grange and Laurent Mortier. 2015. 'Improved overall survival in melanoma with combined dabrafenib and trametinib'. *New England Journal of Medicine* 372(1): 30–39.

Seibel, Nancy L. 2011. 'Using evidence-based programs to support children and families experiencing homelessness'. The National Center on Family Homelessness, National Alliance to End Family Homelessness and ZERO TO THREE.

Shaxson, Louise, Alex Bielak, Ibrahim Ahmed, Derek Brien, Bernadette Conant, Anne Middleton, Catherine Fisher, Elin Gwyn and Laurens Klerkx. 2012. *Expanding Our Understanding of K* (KT, KE, KTT, KMb, KB, KM, etc)*. Hamilton, Ontario: United Nations University, Institute for Water, Environment and Health.

Shepherd, Jonathan. 2007. 'The production and management of evidence for public service reform'. *Evidence & Policy: A Journal of Research, Debate and Practice* 3(2): 231–251.

Slavin, Robert E. 2008. 'Perspectives on evidence-based research in education – what works? Issues in synthesizing educational program evaluations'. *Educational Researcher* 37(1): 5–14. doi: 10.3102/0013189x08314117.

Smith, Adrian. 1996. 'Mad cows and ecstasy: Chance and choice in an evidence-based society'. *Journal of the Royal Statistical Society. Series A (Statistics in Society* 159: 367–384.

Smith, Katherine. 2013. *Beyond Evidence-Based Policy in Public Health: The Interplay of Ideas*. Basingstoke: Palgrave Macmillan.

Starr, Mark, Iain Chalmers, Mike Clarke and Andrew D. Oxman. 2009. 'The origins, evolution and future of the Cochrane Database of Systematic Reviews'. *International Journal of Technology Assessment in Health Care* 51(1): 182–195.

Start, Daniel and Ingie Hovland. 2004. *Tools for Policy Impact: A Handbook for Researchers*. London: Overseas Development Institute.

SUPPORT Programme. undated. *Executive Summary*. Oslo: Nasjonalt kunnskapssenter for helsetjenesten.

Sutcliffe, Sophie and Julius Court. 2005. *Evidence-Based Policymaking: What is it? How Does it Work? What Relevance for Developing Countries?* London: Overseas Development Institute.

Tami Sullivan, Bronwyn Hunter and Bonnie Fisher. 2013. 'Evidence-based policy and practice: The role of the state in advancing criminal justice research. Findings from the Researcher-Practitioner Partnerships Study (RPPS)'. Report presented to the US Department of Justice.

UNCTAD. 2006. *Research-Based Policy Making: Bridging the Gap between Researchers and Policy Makers*. Geneva: United Nations Conference on Trade and Development.

Van der Arend, Jenny. 2014. 'Bridging the research/policy gap: Policy officials' perspectives on the barriers and facilitators to effective links between academic and policy worlds'. *Policy Studies* 35(6): 611–630.

Ward, Vicky, Allan House and Susan Hamer. 2009. 'Knowledge brokering: The missing link in the evidence to action chain?' *Evidence & Policy: A Journal of Research, Debate and Practice* 5(3): 267–279.

Weiss, Carol H. 1979. 'The many meanings of research utilization'. *Public Administration Review* 39(5): 426–431.

——. 1991. 'Policy research: Data, ideas, or arguments'. In *Social Sciences and Modern States: National Experiences and Theoretical Crossroads*, edited by Peter Wagner, Carol

Hirschon Weiss, Björn Wittrock and Hellmut Wollmann, pp. 307–332. Cambridge: Cambridge University Press.

Welsh, Brandon and David Farrington. 2001. 'Toward an evidence-based approach to preventing crime'. *Annals of the American Academy of Political and Social Science* 578(1): 158–173.

Wesselink, Anna, Hal Colebatch and Warren Pearce. 2014. 'Evidence and policy: Discourses, meanings and practices'. *Policy Sciences* 47(4): 339–344. doi: 10.1007/s11077-014-9209-2.

What Works Network. 2014. *What Works? Evidence for Decision Makers*. London: UK Government.

WHO. 2009. *More Research Needed into Childhood Diarrhoea*. Geneva: World Health Organizaion.

——. undated. *EVIPNet: Evidence Informed Policy Network*. Geneva: World Health Organizaion.

Wright, John, Jayne Parry and Jonathan Mathers. 2007. '"What to do about political context?" Evidence synthesis, the New Deal for Communities and the possibilities for evidence-based policy'. *Evidence & Policy: A Journal of Research, Debate and Practice* 3(2): 253–269.

Young, Shaun. 2011. 'Evidence of democracy? The relationship between evidence-based policy and democratic government'. *Journal of Public Administration and Policy Research* 3(1): 19–27.

Part II
The politics of evidence

3 Bias and the politics of evidence

Two forms of bias

Chapter 1 noted the criticisms levelled at the George W. Bush administration for its use of evidence to support the decision to invade Iraq in 2003. Yet the controversy over the war was just one example of the accusations faced over evidence manipulation. The Bush administration was also accused of being 'anti-science' in general, with critics arguing that it routinely ignored evidence that did not align with its ideological positions or that it deliberately invented or manipulated scientific evidence to suit political goals (cf. Duncan 2007; Mooney 2006). This led, at the time, for the non-profit Union of Concerned Scientists to state: 'There is a well-established pattern of suppression and distortion of scientific findings', concluding that the administration was manipulating science to 'an unprecedented degree' (2004, p. 28).

Bush's successor, Barack Obama, presumably laid out a different approach in his 2009 inaugural address when he stated:

> The question we ask today is not whether our government is too big or too small, but whether it works – whether it helps families find jobs at a decent wage, care they can afford, a retirement that is dignified. Where the answer is yes, we intend to move forward. Where the answer is no, programs will end. And those of us who manage the public's dollars will be held to account, to spend wisely, reform bad habits, and do our business in the light of day, because only then can we restore the vital trust between a people and their government.
>
> (White House 2009)

Obama's invocation of the 'what works' language could be seen in many ways as a rebuke of Bush's approach, but the quote also illustrates the powerful ideas that appropriate use of evidence can better achieve social goals and, further, can be a critical requirement for trust in a democratic society.

Obama's apparent embrace of evidence has not gone unnoticed. One British charity claimed that: 'President Barack Obama and his administration have developed and are now implementing the most extensive evidence-based initiatives in US history' (Haskins and Baron 2011, p. 4). And yet, despite this, the Obama administration has not been without its own controversies around evidence use. In 2013, for example, the President was criticised over a policy decision to impose a minimum age restriction of 15 years for access to emergency contraception (the so-called 'morning after pill' or 'Plan B'), even though the US Food and Drug Administration (FDA) stated that the pill was safe and effective for girls of all ages. According to one critical commentator: 'the Obama administration stepped in to overrule the FDA – a political overreach that wasn't based on the scientific evidence, but rather [signalled] a decision to disregard it' (Culp-Ressler 2013). Eventually a US District Court ordered the Obama administration to make the contraception available to younger individuals, claiming that the age restriction was 'politically motivated' and 'scientifically unjustified' (Dennis and Kliff 2013).

So what does this tell us when 'politically motivated' decisions can come from multiple sides of the political spectrum? In fact, the emergency contraception case highlights three fundamental, but distinct, challenges related to the politics of evidence. The first has to do with the concerns of evidence advocates over the ways in which pieces of evidence can be misused in unscientific ways for political purposes. In the emergency contraception case, this can be illustrated when the White House defended the age limit by stating that '[the contraception] could be dangerous if misused' (White House Office of the Press Secretary 2013) – a statement that appears to exaggerate the risks, considering it was judged no more harmful than other drugs available to teenagers without a prescription (e.g. non-prescription painkillers).

The second fundamental challenge has to deal with whether clinical evidence – in this case evidence about the safety and effectiveness of the morning after pill – should be the *only* criteria on which to base a decision to provide it. Those in favour of an age restriction on emergency contraception typically do so because they have concerns about governmental involvement in decisions that they feel should involve parents. Just because the contraception is safe for 14 year olds, there is still disagreement as to whether or not a government should make it readily available to 14 year olds without parental notification. Whatever one's position on state versus parental responsibility, what is important here is to recognise that *this is a decidedly political question* with multiple issues to consider. Yet a court explicitly ruled that the decision *could not be political* and that the contraception should be provided based on evidence of safety alone. However, justifying this position by reference to scientific evidence appears to obscure and exclude the other relevant social concerns from the decision-making process.

Seen in this way, *technical bias* relates to problematic uses of evidence from the perspective of scientific best practice. In political settings, evidence advocates see it as a particular problem when evidence is misused to serve political goals – what might be considered the *politicisation of science. Issue bias*, however, reflects the ways in which the invocation of particular forms of evidence can obscure the political nature of decisions and, in doing so, 'bias' decisions towards particular outcomes – what can be described as the *depoliticisation of politics.* The fact that a choice of evidence can influence decisions is not necessarily a problem in and of itself – as policymaking fundamentally requires information to help value or measure various options. Yet it is important to recognise whether particular pieces (or uses) of evidence work to shift policy priority to one set of values over another. So while policy scholars would argue that choice between values is in many ways the nature of decision making, *issue bias* can be seen as problematic if it obscures or undermines the explicit consideration of the multiple sets of values that are important to the public (see similar points made in Barnes and Parkhurst 2014; Russell et al. 2008).

If issue bias systematically arises through practices or norms that routinely privilege particular types of evidence, it can further be understood as an exercise in political power. This interpretation reflects the work of political scientists Peter Bachrach and Morton Baratz, who studied power outside traditional decision-making processes such as legislative voting or elections. The authors coined the term 'mobilization of bias' specifically to refer to how power can be exercised through: '[a] set of predominant values, beliefs, rituals, and institutional procedures ("rules of the game") that operate systematically and consistently to the benefit of certain persons and groups at the expense of others' (Bachrach and Baratz 1970, p. 43). Promotion of particular norms of evidence use can do just this – working to set these rules of the game in policy decisions informed by evidence – and champions of EBP must be aware of the political implications of doing so.

Returning to the emergency contraception example, it is worth noting that the US presidency is a decidedly political role, tasked with representing the public's views and values as such. The FDA, on the other hand, is a technical agency tasked with the regulation and provision of expert advice on issues of public health, while the courts are judicial bodies tasked with overseeing or hearing challenges about the legality of particular policy decisions. It is also worth recognising that the US Constitution provides many of the rules by which these branches of government interact, and determines when and how courts can over-rule the executive. In other countries with differing governance arrangements, there will naturally be differences in how evidence is brought to bear in political decision making and the roles that courts or technical agencies can play.[1]

In the emergency contraception case, a court ruled that a social policy decision must not be 'politically motivated'. But while this may have been done under the rubric of embracing evidence, the political result was that the court effectively took two social concerns – safety and effectiveness – and ruled that these alone should be the basis of the decision, thereby forcing the administration to disregard any other political concerns (such as parental involvement for contraceptive choices of minors). When viewed from a *technical* perspective, the administration's claims that it might be 'dangerous' for youth to have access to the drugs

1 More on the governing arrangements shaping evidence use is discussed in Chapters 7 and 8, and interested readers can see the work of Jasanoff (1987, 2006) for greater exploration of how political cultures and constitutional structures affect science policymaking.

appears to be biased, but viewed from a *political* perspective, the court appears to have made a decision over which social values to prioritise, introducing a different form of bias over the issues considered.

However, a third key challenge that this example illustrates is the question of whether it is within the authority of the courts to make such a decision in the first place. This reflects a concern with the *legitimacy of the process* through which evidence is used – which includes issues of *who* should be making the decisions over which evidence to use and *when* particular forms of evidence should determine policy decisions. This chapter begins our exploration of the politics of evidence by exploring the nature of both technical bias and issue bias. The following chapters will investigate the origins and mechanisms by which those forms of bias arise. Subsequently, the final section of the book will discuss the systems that govern evidence use, which includes consideration of the legitimacy of the evidence-to-policy process.

Technical bias

The previous chapter noted that one of the biggest challenges to the EBP movement is how it has typically assumed that evidence can have specific and direct implications to inform policy action. This reflects what Carol Weiss (1979) has described as a 'problem-solving' role for research (more recently described as 'instrumental' use in Weiss 1998). However, as detailed in Chapter 2, Weiss is widely cited for having described a number of other ways in which research influences policy, noting that the problem-solving role of research will only be relevant to a fairly limited number of cases where there is already agreement on policy goals (Weiss 1979). For years, Weiss' framework has been applied to critique the idea that evidence can simply tell us 'what works' to solve policy problems. Yet even with this limitation in mind, there remain a number of valid concerns about the problematic uses of evidence voiced by EBP advocates. Indeed, while evidence may not tell us what is the right thing to do at all times, there are still more or less valid ways to use evidence. Pieces of evidence can be scientifically robust or they can be methodologically flawed. Findings from research can be interpreted in ways that are true to their methods or that are inconsistent with their conclusions. And bodies of evidence can be reviewed rigorously or cherry-picked strategically. All of these examples of poorer practice can genuinely be problems for policymaking, and the set of ways in which scientific best practices are contravened provides the overarching conceptualisation of what is referred to here as technical bias.

However, technically biased uses of evidence can actually take a number of forms, and in the following we highlight three particular stages where these can arise: in the *creation* of evidence, in the *selection* of evidence and in the *interpretation* of evidence. Distinguishing these is not only important in helping us identify and classify instances of technical bias, but it can also be useful to help explore the various origins of bias and, as such, to guide efforts aiming to reduce its incidence or impact (this is explored in greater depth in Chapters 4 and 5).

Technical bias in the creation of evidence

In some cases, research evidence may be judged as biased simply due to the way in which it was created. According to established ideas of good scientific practice, research should be conducted from an impartial position, designed to test hypotheses or create new ones, without any personal or political goal influencing the research design (Begley 2013; Douglas 2015). Yet we can see numerous cases where policy-relevant research is undertaken in ways that are structured to provide a particular answer or are strategically manipulated to produce desired outputs. Some of the most obvious examples of this can be seen when corporations or private sector actors have undertaken research designed to produce favourable results to support their products. In their 2001 book, Rampton and Stauber provide a sweeping depiction of the ways in which industry actors manipulate science and research for their own interests. They argue that there is a 'systemwide bias that industry funding creates among researchers in commercially profitable fields', further noting that 'a host of techniques exist for manipulating research protocols to produce studies whose conclusions fit their sponsor's predetermined interests' (2001, p. 217).

One corporate sector particularly renowned for its manipulation of research has been the tobacco industry. In 1998, a landmark court case in the US state of Minnesota forced six tobacco companies to place millions of pages of internal documents and correspondence in publicly accessible repositories for a period of ten years (Hurt et al. 2009). A number of studies were subsequently conducted to analyse these documents, revealing a range of strategies taken by tobacco companies to create and manipulate research evidence in order to deliberately mislead the public on the harms of smoking (Bero 2005; Cummings, Brown and O'Connor 2007). In one example, Wertz and colleagues (2011) found evidence showing how the Phillip Morris company undertook research on the harmful effects of cigarette flavour additives, revealing that the company adjusted its data and changed its study protocols after initial statistical findings showed harmful effects. The authors claim that the company specifically designed studies to be underpowered to reduce the number of significant findings that could arise. In another case, Tong and Glantz (2007) describe 'design bias' in industry-sponsored research that looked at whether spouses of smokers had higher rates of heart disease. By strategically choosing how exposure was defined, the research found no statistical association between second-hand smoke and heart disease.

The tobacco industry example is perhaps the most striking because it is a clear case of where an industry has produced a product known for years to be harmful (Cummings, Brown and O'Connor 2007), but deliberately undertook research designed to sow doubt about this in order to resist policies of regulation. Yet strategic creation of evidence is not unique to this case. Rampton and Stauber (2001) and Goldacre (2014) have both accused the pharmaceutical industry, for example, of strategically manipulating research to produce favourable results or to hide unfavourable results in order to maximise their profits. In theory, pharmaceuticals are designed to be beneficial to health, and new drugs should be rigorously tested to ensure they are more beneficial than other alternatives. Yet Goldacre argues: 'Drugs are tested by the people who manufacture them, in poorly designed trials, on hopelessly small numbers of weird, unrepresentative patients, and analysed using techniques which are flawed by design, in such a way that they exaggerate the benefits of treatments' (2014, p. xi) Such claims may appear bold, but they appear to have some empirical validation. Fries and Krishnan (2004), for example, conducted a study which analysed research presented to a rheumatology conference. They looked to see whether drug trials supported by industry funding were more likely to show positive results, finding that 100 per cent of the included studies funded by the industry were positive. The authors concluded that it was not simply selection bias, whereby favourable studies were presented at the conference, but also design bias, indicating that the trials themselves may have been specifically constructed to produce these results. This finding corresponds to other reviews that have consistently found that industry sponsorship of drug research increases the likelihood of positive findings being reported (Bekelman, Li and Gross 2003, Lundh et al. 2012).

Another example that has appeared in popular media can be seen in the case of the anti-depressant drug paroxetine – sold as *Paxil* by the company GlaxoSmithKline. According to news-magazine *The Economist*: 'By the early 2000s [*Paxil*] was earning the firm nearly $2billion a year. It was being prescribed to millions of children and teenagers on the basis of a trial, called Study 329, which suggested it was a good treatment for depressed youngsters' (2016, p. 82). Yet according to a 2015 re-analysis of the trial data, the drug had actually showed no significant improvements over placebo in all its primary or secondary outcomes of interest (Le Noury et al. 2015). Rather, GlaxoSmithKline has been accused of 'outcome switching' in which researchers kept looking for new outcomes mid-trial to find something to show statistically significant results, which were then published as if they were the original goals all along (*The Economist* 2016). However, also particularly worryingly in this case was an apparent miscoding of serious suicide attempts in the trial, making the drug appear no more risky than placebo when, in fact, it may have increased suicidal episodes (Le Noury et al. 2015). While the company has not admitted liability, articles describing the case paint a picture of a drug company manipulating data to make billions of dollars from a drug that is no more beneficial than placebo, but that potentially increased the risk of attempted suicide amongst millions of depressed young persons for more than a decade. The case led to the largest ever regulatory fine of a pharmaceutical company in the US (US$3 billion) and led one journalist to comment that this case 'appears to be a direct demonstration of how a company and researchers can misinterpret the data to make a bad drug look good' (Dobbs 2015).

Yet it is not only corporate actors who may create evidence in biased ways. There have always been cases of individual scientists undertaking flawed research or following unscientific practices as well – driven by career ambitions, financial interests, or ideological goals. Indeed, one systematic review found that, in anonymous surveys, nearly 2 per cent of scientists admitted having ever falsified data, with nearly 34 per cent admitting other forms of research misconduct such as 'modifying results' to improve outcomes (Fanelli 2009). There can even be entire fields of research that are controversial and judged as technically biased by the nature of their approach. 'Creation research', for example, is a body of work that has grown in recent years (particularly in the US) that seeks to provide evidence that supports the belief that the earth was created by a divine power a few thousand years ago (the 'young earth' hypothesis). However, this field of work has been criticised as fundamentally flawed, in part due to its explicit goal to prove a pre-determined position – that is, to prove biblical literalism – rather than to use evidence without prejudgement (Pigliucci 2002).

Technical bias in the selection of evidence

While the above cases illustrate how the research process can be manipulated to *create* biased evidence, technical bias can also occur in the *selection* of evidence, when a body of (potentially technically valid) evidence is cherry-picked so as to only highlight those pieces of evidence which support a desired outcome. This is particularly a problem in policy debates touching on complex or uncertain issues, as in such situations there can be many pieces of relevant information, and such information may be contradictory. Indeed, it is very rare to have all evidence and all studies showing the same outcomes or the same direction of effect in any scientific field of enquiry. Often there is a range of findings, and it is necessary to look at the totality of the evidence to discern a pattern or overall trend. This is frequently why systematic reviews of research are so important in the EBP field, as they aim to follow explicit steps to ensure that all relevant evidence is considered. Yet in contested political debates, we often see the opposite occurring. The selective use of pieces of evidence allows groups to focus on different facts in line with their political needs and goals.

Biased selection of evidence is perhaps no more apparent than in the debates over climate change, where accusations of cherry-picking have appeared on all sides of the policy spectrum. The Institute of Climate Studies, for instance, has argued that global warming sceptics cherry-pick data to select limited range time periods of eight, ten or 12 years that might show no increase in global surface temperature, yet it argues if one includes all data from 1970 to the present day, a very clear increasing trend can be seen (Institute of Climate Studies 2013). Alternatively, in a post for the 'Global Warming Policy Forum' (an organisation that defines itself as sceptical of climate change data), Whitehouse (2014) makes almost the identical critique of the Committee on Climate Change, claiming it cherry-picked data by choosing start years for a trend analysis which over-emphasise increasing temperature trends. In effect, both sides are accusing each other of the same strategy to select evidence in technically biased ways.

There are, of course, more or less systematic and robust ways to interpret climate data, and a number of professional scientific bodies have put their voice behind claims that climate change is indeed real (cf. Joint Academies of Science undated). Yet it is not only complex problems such as this that can demonstrate biased selection of evidence. The same can also be seen in more mundane cases and, indeed, may be a routine approach taken by policymakers at times. The oft-lamented concept of 'policy-based evidence making', for instance, captures the way that politicians have (at times) actively called for evidence to support pre-existing policy plans or ideas. The Chief Scientific Officer to the European Commission, Professor Anne Glover, specifically criticised this phenomenon when, speaking in 2014, she stated: 'Let's imagine a Commissioner over the weekend thinks, "Let's ban the use of credit cards in the EU because credit cards lead to personal debt". So that commissioner will come in on Monday morning and say to his or her Director General, "Find me the evidence that demonstrates that this is the case"' (EurActive.com 2014).

While Professor Glover presented a hypothetical case, one does not need to look far to find examples of political officials accused of doing this in practice. Chapter 1 discussed the case of the George W. Bush administration being criticised for apparently cherry-picking or manipulating evidence to justify the 2003 Iraq war (cf. Hersh 2003; Pillar 2006; Van der Heide 2013). The administration was also accused of selective uses of evidence and the appointment of biased advisors to justify policy positions on issues ranging from sexual health to environmental protection (Gordon, Smyth and Diehl 2008; Union of Concerned Scientists 2004).

Clearly, it is not just in the US that this can occur. In the UK, for instance, the Labour government of 1997–2010 explicitly embraced the language of evidence, famously stating in its party manifesto that 'what counts is what works'. Yet even under this rhetorical banner to embrace evidence, a report of the House of Commons Select Committee on Science and Technology found that civil servants serving the Labour government were ignoring data that did not suit policy objectives (Giles 2006). The report gives a particularly poignant example of how commissioned research by civil servants could illustrate both biased creation and selection of evidence, stating:

> we were extremely concerned to hear allegations from certain academics that departments have been commissioning and publishing research selectively in order to 'prop up' policies. Professor Tim Hope, a criminologist from the University of Keele who has worked with the Home Office, told us: 'it was with sadness and regret that I saw our work ill-used and our faith in government's use of evidence traduced'. Of two case studies looking at burglary reduction commissioned by the Home Office, Professor Hope told us that the department decided to only write up one: 'Presumably . . . because the area-wide reduction was greater here than elsewhere.' Professor Hope also accused the Home Office of manipulating the data so as 'to capitalise on chance, producing much more favourable findings overall', despite the fact

> that 'for individual projects, the [Home Office] method produces considerable distortion'. Furthermore, Professor Hope alleged that the Home Office had interfered with presentation of research findings by other researchers.
>
> (House of Commons Science and Technology Committee 2006, pp. 49–50)

Strategic uses of evidence and 'policy-based evidence making' can therefore be seen as a problem cutting across party ideologies and national borders alike.

Technical bias in the interpretation of evidence

The third way in which technical bias can arise is in the interpretation of evidence, whereby invalid conclusions are drawn from an otherwise comprehensive body of existing data or evidence. More simply, this would reflect cases where evidence is taken to say something that it, in fact, does not.

Correlations interpreted as causal

Such errors are incredibly widespread and do not necessarily have political origins. We seem to need constant reminding, for instance, that 'correlation does not equate

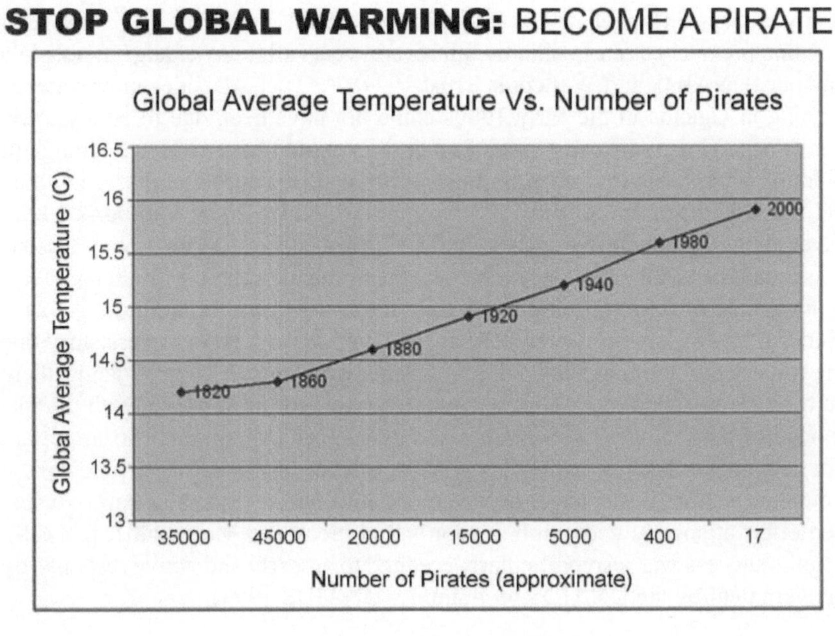

Figure 3.1 Correlation does not mean causality: example.

Source: Obtained from http://www.venganza.org/images/spreadword/pchart1.pdf, reproduced with permission.

to causality' – as it is so common that individuals make this error of interpretation. Indeed, a widely distributed graph developed by the 'Church of the Flying Spaghetti Monster' serves as a reminder of the fallacy of assuming causality, as it illustrates that average global temperature shows a strong statistically significant correlation with falls in the global number of pirates since the early nineteenth century.[2]

This is a humorous example, yet inaccurate causal assumptions can have very real consequences in public policy realms. One example of this can be seen in the field of HIV/AIDS prevention. Throughout the 1980s and 1990s, AIDS grew to be one the biggest causes of premature death in Africa and one of its greatest development challenges. As such, there has been a tremendous amount of work undertaken to try to understand how to prevent the spread of HIV, along with searches for examples of 'what works' for HIV prevention. In the 1990s and 2000s, the two most famous cases of HIV success in Africa were Uganda and Senegal – Uganda for being the only African nation to see falling HIV prevalence over time and Senegal for keeping its HIV rates low in the first place. As such, it has been natural to look to these countries for lessons of success, but some of the resultant claims in these cases have been shown to be based on incorrect assumptions of causality (Parkhurst 2013).

In the early years of Uganda's success, for instance, claims were often made that it was particular programmes of the government, such as the national 'multisectoral approach' launched in 1993, that explained the falling HIV rates of the 1990s. This helped support a rapid emulation of this approach elsewhere, with multisectoral HIV/AIDS programmes being particularly popular in the 1990s and early 2000s in many countries (Putzel 2004). Yet epidemiological models of HIV show that population prevalence rates will only fall several years after any change in people's behaviour (UNAIDS and Wellcome Trust 1999). As such, declines in prevalence beginning in Uganda in the early 1990s could not have been due to policy interventions occurring at the same time. Rather, they would have reflected a range of population-wide behaviour changes that occurred several years earlier – i.e. they could not have been due to the 1993 programme (Kirby 2008; Parkhurst 2002). So even though Uganda saw falls in its HIV prevalence rates, the policy lessons learned could be technically inaccurate when temporal correlations (policies occurring at the time of prevalence falls) were assumed to be causal (Parkhurst 2002).

Senegal has widely been presented as the other African HIV success story due to the country maintaining a low HIV prevalence over time. As with Uganda, there have been claims about the policy actions that 'worked' in this case, with the former head of the UNAIDS programme and colleagues explaining: 'An important factor in Senegal's success at keeping HIV prevalence low, contrary to much of the surrounding region, is the active involvement of religious leaders as part of a sustained effort at society wide mobilization' (Piot, Seck and Marie 2001, p. 1108). Senegal's success was also particularly credited to an early and active response by the government by the UNAIDS programme (UNAIDS 1999).

2 Many other 'spurious correlations' can be seen in a book by Vigen (2015), including how bedsheet suffocation and strangulation deaths are highly correlated with US cheese consumption, and accidental swimming pool drownings are correlated with the number of films made by actor Nicolas Cage.

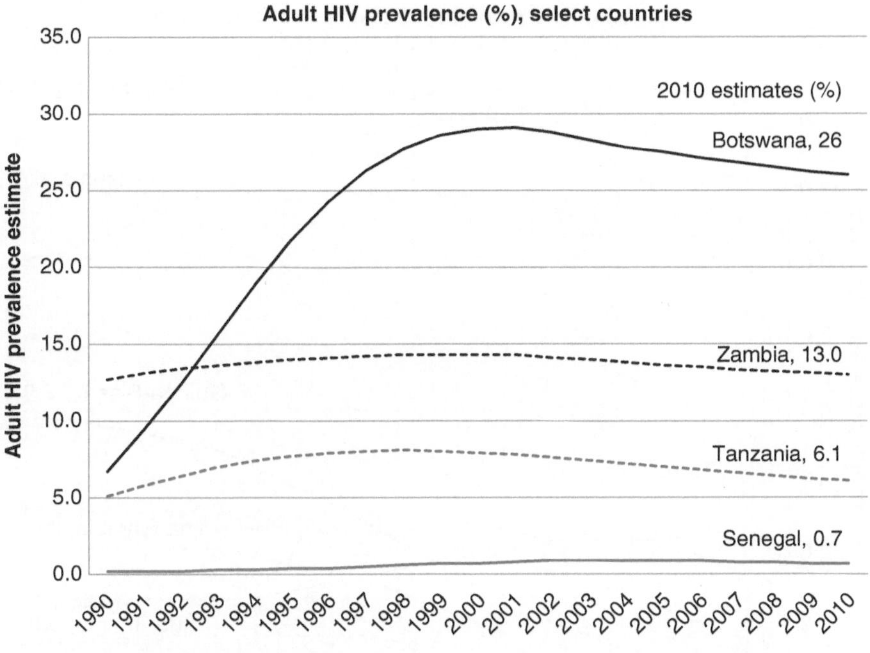

Figure 3.2 Senegal's HIV prevalence over time compared to other select countries.

Source: Based on data from www.unaids.org/en/dataanalysis/datatools; figure updated and adapted from Parkhurst (2013).

If we look more specifically at the Senegalese data, we can indeed see how it appears particularly remarkable if compared to some of the other countries in Sub-Saharan Africa facing much larger HIV epidemics. Figure 3.2. below illustrates this, comparing Senegal's HIV prevalence over time to a set of higher-prevalence countries.

Comparing Senegal to countries such as Botswana, Tanzania and Zambia would naturally give the impression that it must have done something that 'works' – and the early and inclusive political response from the Senegalese government would be a natural explanation as the cause. Unfortunately, a comparison such as that presented in Figure 3.2 would reflect a technically biased interpretation of the data based on an incorrect counterfactual. The assumption implied in this figure, and within the statement of Piot and colleagues quoted above, is that HIV rates would naturally have been much higher. However, none of these African countries with very high HIV prevalence are anywhere near Senegal geographically. Senegal is located in West Africa, while the highest HIV rates on the continent have occurred in East and Southern Africa. If we instead compare Senegal's HIV prevalence to the countries that border Senegal (which did not have notable early or widespread political responses), we see that

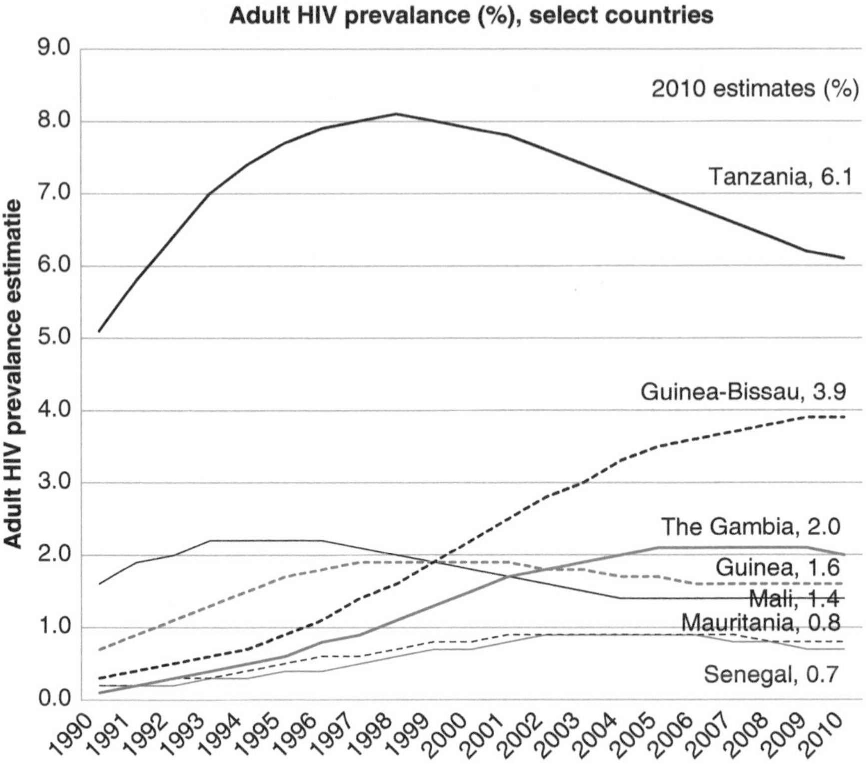

Figure 3.3 Senegal's HIV prevalence over time compared to its neighbours.

Source: Based on data from www.unaids.org/en/dataanalysis/datatools; figure updated and adapted from Parkhurst (2013).

most of these countries also had low HIV prevalence and one (Mauritania) had almost identical prevalence to Senegal.

This figure gives a much more realistic presentation of Senegal's success. It illustrates that while Senegal did indeed see low prevalence rates, there is simply not a lot of HIV in that part of West Africa. Tanzania is shown for comparison, but it lies almost 6,000 km away from Senegal, slightly farther than the distance from Senegal to Iceland. Senegal and neighbouring Mauritania, on the other hand, had nearly identical prevalence rates over this period. Guinea-Bissau shows the highest levels of the group, but it is also worth noting that these data are estimates as of 2016. In fact, when many claims of Senegal's success were being made, the estimates of most of its neighbours were significantly lower, which would give even less reason to think that Senegal was successful at the time (e.g. a UNAIDS document on Senegal's success was published in 1999, when none of Senegal's neighbours experienced HIV prevalence higher than 2 per cent). Compared to most of its neighbours, Senegal does have slightly lower HIV prevalence in the early years, but these differences are reasonably small – and it makes it harder to hold Senegal's political response as a strong example of 'what works' in African HIV prevention, as has often been done (cf. UNAIDS 2012).

Misinterpreting risk statistics

Another example of biased interpretation of evidence that can have important policy implications is in the misunderstanding of risk statistics. A particularly persistent example of this can be seen in the regular confusion between *absolute risk* and *relative risk* of an outcome occurring. Absolute risk is the chance of something actually happening, while relative risk is the difference in the chances of it occurring between two comparison situations. Members of the public may not be so clear on this distinction, and while research studies often report relative risk in their findings, media coverage of research findings can often be unclear. So, for example, a recent news story reported that people who drink one sugar-sweetened beverage per day have 'an 18 percent increased risk of developing [Type 2 diabetes] over a decade' (Aubrey 2015). This does not mean that 18 per cent of the people who drink these beverages will contract diabetes; rather, it means that the *chance* of contracting diabetes was 18 per cent higher (Imamura et al. 2015). If someone already had a 10 per cent chance (absolute risk) of contracting Type 2 diabetes, then the daily drinking of sugar-sweetened beverages would raise their absolute risk to 11.8 per cent (11.8 per cent being 18 per cent higher than 10 per cent).

However, confusion in risk statistics can be critical for policymaking, as the perceived chance of something occurring is particularly important to help decide the political priority of an issue. If a condition is very rare, then a large increase in relative risk still may not actually warrant a high priority policy response – e.g. if we imagine we have a one-in-a-million chance of contracting a rare life-threatening disease, this is a risk of 0.0001 per cent. A news story that reports on a 50 per cent increase in risk might sound dramatic, but if that were the relative increase, it would mean our absolute risk of contracting the disease rises to 0.00015 per cent – or one-and-a-half-in-a-million. We would then justifiably need to ask if such a change warrants significant policy attention.

It is unfortunately common to see no distinction between relative and absolute risk, even though the implications can be huge for how important the issue is for public action. Indeed, at times we are simply told that something 'increases risk', without specifying either the relative or absolute figures. An example of this can be seen when the UK's *BBC News* reported that there was 'cancer risk even from light drinking' (Roberts 2015), giving no specific figures on the risk levels involved. The article did link to the original research (see Cao et al. 2015), but without any indication of the relative and/or absolute risks involved, a headline about alcohol leading to cancer risk serves simply to invoke an emotional reaction and prohibits an informed analysis of the actual situation, perpetuating ignorance or confusion over the various meanings of 'risk'.

There are of course a number of other ways in which evidence can be interpreted in a technically biased fashion. Non-significant statistical findings may be understood incorrectly as if they are somehow significant. Alternatively, results that do show statistical significance may be assumed to represent 'fact' when the result still could be due to chance. Indeed, if a research study does many tests on its data at a 5 per cent level of significance, one would still expect one out of 20 such tests to show significance through random chance alone. However, the use of technically biased evidence, of all the kinds discussed, can have obvious negative implications for policymaking. It can mislead the public, it can serve to promote the interests of powerful groups controlling information and it can result in less effective or potentially harmful policy choices than if technically valid evidence were utilised. These are fundamental concerns within the EBP movement in their calls to improve evidence use and, given the frequency of technical bias, there is good reason for such concerns.

Issue bias

A second form of bias to consider, however, is that of issue bias. Albert Einstein is often quoted as having said 'not everything that can be counted counts, and not everything that counts can be counted'. Unfortunately, this seems to be an incorrect attribution,[3] as the quote actually appears to come from sociologist William Cameron, who wrote:

> It would be nice if all of the data which sociologists require could be enumerated because then we could run them through IBM machines and draw charts as the economists do. However, *not everything that can be counted counts, and not everything that counts can be counted.*
>
> (Cameron 1963, p. 13, emphasis added)

Such an error in attribution could be seen as an example of technical bias. It is *technically* incorrect if we say that Einstein was the origin of this expression. But the implication of the quote, regardless of who said it, takes us to the heart of *issue bias*. Fundamentally, calls for policy to *follow* or be *based on* particular forms of evidence risk insisting that policy be directed based on what has been counted, not necessarily what counts. However, issue bias can also manifest itself in different ways – in either the creation, the selection or the interpretation of evidence.

Issue bias in the creation of evidence

As with technical bias, the first manifestation of issue bias can be in the creation of evidence itself. Nancy Krieger, a social epidemiologist, has noted that: 'If you don't ask, you don't know, and if you don't know, you can't act' (1992, p. 412) – fundamentally capturing the importance that the choice of research question can

3 See http://quoteinvestigator.com/2010/05/26/everything-counts-einstein.

have in shaping future policy action alternatives. In contrast to the previous concern over scientifically flawed research design, then, this section reflects on how choices made over what issues to research, how to study them and what questions to ask within a study can have political implications, even if the research is conducted in rigorous and valid ways.

Generating evidence through research takes time and money, both of which are finite. As such, the choice of what social issues to study requires some level of prioritisation or selection between alternatives. Decisions over when and where to do research will, accordingly, be a fundamentally value-based exercise, even if it is not commonly discussed in such terms (Douglas 2015). In the field of global health, for instance, there is increasing concern about so-called 'neglected tropical diseases' that afflict poorer parts of the world which have not received nearly as much attention (from governments and billionaire philanthropists alike) as the 'big three' of HIV, tuberculosis and malaria (Hotez and Kamath 2009; Remme et al. 2002). If global health policy were simply to follow evidence of 'what works', then policies addressing malaria, tuberculosis or HIV would clearly dominate political agendas and neglected diseases would remain neglected simply because those controlling research funds have not yet made efforts to conduct investigations on these diseases.

There is also typically a dearth of evidence about the social needs of hidden or so-called marginalised populations in various settings. In some cases, there may be a deliberate societal bias against studying the needs of a particular group. Ethnic minorities, the poor, immigrants, the homeless or other stigmatised groups may face systemic discrimination, which means that they are less likely to be the subject of research in the first place. There may also be groups in great need of policy attention, but for whom evidence generation is nearly impossible. Research on victims of human trafficking, for example, is plagued by challenges due to the hidden and illegal nature of the subject (Di Nicola 2007; Tyldum and Brunovskis 2005). If political choices or agendas were driven exclusively by availability of evidence about a problem, this would result in issue bias in the ways in which the specific needs of these groups were excluded from attention.

Even when a topic is being investigated, issue bias can still arise from the choice of which outcomes to measure within the evaluation of a project or programme, as the selection of outcomes serves as a de facto indication of what 'success' looks like and hence what social values are seen to be important. The emergency contraception case above provides one example. The FDA in this instance was mandated to evaluate drug safety and effectiveness, but not social acceptability. But, as shown, in practice this meant that the evidence base only incorporated some of the potentially relevant social concerns. A similar example can be seen in the evaluation of harm reduction programmes to assist individuals who inject illegal drugs. Supporters of harm reduction typically see drug users as ill and in need of treatment, and are primarily concerned with health risks such as overdoses or the spread of infections like HIV from needle sharing. Opponents, on the other hand, often see drug users as criminals and typically are concerned that harm reduction sends the 'wrong message' about drugs or diverts funds from other preferred strategies (like programmes to arrest drug sellers or to stop the initiation of drug use in the first place). Given the differences of values at stake, the choice of how to evaluate harm reduction programmes can, in effect, indicate which social concerns are deemed to be important and, as such, can introduce issue bias if outcomes of interest to only one side of the debate are included.

Such a situation can be seen in the evaluation of a Canadian harm reduction programme called InSite, which provided safe injecting sites and access to medical care for drug users in Vancouver. Harm reduction was controversial in Canada at the time, with the conservative Prime Minister Stephen Harper saying in 2006 that he was 'philosophically opposed to safe-injection sites but would wait for evidence of InSite's effectiveness before making a decision' (*Ottawa Citizen* 2006). An evaluation of the programme was indeed conducted, finding that InSite had 'an array of community and public health benefits' (Wood et al. 2006, p. 1399), including reduced needle sharing and decreased public discarding of needles. This led to the Canadian Supreme Court to rule in 2011 that the clinic was not in violation of drug laws and should stay open, arguing: 'InSite saves lives. Its benefits have been proven' (*CBC News* 2011).

So does that mean that Prime Minister Harper embraced the ruling of the Supreme Court as 'evidence-based'? Perhaps unsurprisingly, this was not the case. Harper's response was instead to state: 'I'm disappointed . . . The preference of this government in dealing with drug crime is obviously to prosecute those who sell drugs and create drug addiction in our population and in our youth' (MacQueen and Patriquin 2011).

Advocates of EBP might throw their hands up and see this as an example of politics 'ignoring' evidence. Yet what is critical to recognise is that in the programme evaluation, a choice was made to measure needle sharing, overdoses and publicly discarded needles, but *not to measure* things like whether InSite has an overall impact on 'drug crime' (presumably selling of drugs) or the cost-effectiveness of InSite in comparison to interventions to increase prosecution of drug sellers. As in the case of the morning after pill in the US, it was a court that judged on the legitimacy of a programme, citing the scientific evidence base to do so – yet also as in the US case, the scientific evidence base only measured some of the concerns that were being debated.

Issue bias in the selection of evidence

Issue bias can also be introduced in the selection of evidence, when a supposedly 'evidence-based' argument is made by reference to the bodies of evidence that only represent a limited number of relevant social concerns. Indeed, while EBP advocates often speak as if evidence can somehow overcome political divisions, when a policy can have multiple social impacts and outcomes, then groups on both sides of a political debate can make claims that their preferred solution is 'evidence-based' simply by choosing different outcomes of interest.

A simple hypothetical example of this can be reflected in an infrastructure project, such as building an additional airport runway to increase capacity. There may be a robust (and presumably technically valid) evidence base about the economic growth that is associated with such projects. There may also be a robust (and also technically valid) evidence base about the noise or environmental harms that these projects also engender. Therefore, supporters and opponents of the programme can both appeal to facts to support their case, both making claims that their policy choices are 'evidence-based'.

A real-life example can be seen in the seemingly intractable debates over gun control in the US, which has been a highly charged political topic for decades (Bruce-Briggs 1976; Kleck 1986). However, it is difficult to identify any obvious 'evidence-based gun control policy' due to the fact that there are many social concerns raised within these debates. There is no single right answer on whether gun control laws should address how armed citizens behave, how armed criminals behave, accidental deaths, social attitudes towards violence, the public's views of gun rights, jobs or tax revenue arising from gun ownership, or the host of other concerns that are at times raised by debates over gun control laws. As such, the use of evaluation evidence can clearly have policy implications simply based on which outcomes were evaluated. If one reviews evaluations of how criminals behave in relation to armed citizens or whether being armed affects how much victims lose during a theft (cf. Kleck 1986; Southwick 2000), this would support policies of gun liberalisation. Alternatively, if one reviews the studies that evaluate the risk of death from the widespread availability of guns (cf. Burger 2002; Leenaars and Lester 1997), this evidence base would alternatively support policy positions for greater control. These bodies of evidence may be used systematically and in technically valid ways, but they impose issue bias if claims are made for an 'evidence-based gun policy' when only some social concerns are considered.

Issue bias in the interpretation of evidence

Erroneous interpretations of findings would usually represent examples of technical bias. However, in theory, there can also be cases where a piece of evidence is incorrectly interpreted in a way that prioritises a particular social outcome to the exclusion of others. If a programme evaluation spoke to multiple social concerns, for example – perhaps considering costs, environmental impact, public interest and economic growth – but was incorrectly interpreted as only speaking to some of those outcomes, this might be such a case.

Issue bias and the prioritisation of randomised controlled trials and evidence hierarchies

More relevant, however, is how the concept of issue bias captures the problematic idea that evidence generated by randomised controlled trials (RCTs), (or from the top of particular hierarchies) should be prioritised to inform policy decisions. As noted in the previous chapter, RCTs are fundamentally designed to measure intervention effect, but they do not necessarily indicate the value of what is measured from a policy perspective. The prioritisation of particular forms of evidence based on their methodological features is, in effect, interpreting methodological rigour as a measure of policy relevance. This can therefore generate issue bias if it leads to a de facto policy priority for those concerns for which there have been attempts to undertake RCTs or for policy solutions that are conducive to RCTs (Barnes and Parkhurst 2014).

The previous chapter gave the example of the robust evidence on the effectiveness of Sildenafil (*Viagra*) not necessarily equating to the social importance of the provision of that treatment. Yet the health sector, which particularly embraces RCTs, illustrates a range of other cases where deference to hierarchies of evidence might lead to issue bias. One example is in the ongoing health debates about how much to focus on prevention versus treatment of health problems. Medical treatments are typically much more conducive to testing in RCTs – with all new pharmaceuticals and surgical interventions typically evaluated in this way. However, prevention efforts may be much harder to evaluate experimentally, especially when they aim to address broader social or structural determinants of ill health. In such cases, causal links are less direct, individuals can rarely be isolated from populations, and interventions may work differently in different settings. So while it may be conceptually simple to undertake an experiment to test the efficacy of bypass surgery or stents for heart disease (cf. Cohen et al. 2011), it may be much harder to test experimentally social interventions aiming to reduce heart disease in a population through increased exercise or improved nutrition, for example. It is not *impossible* to undertake social experiments that address disease-related factors such as obesity (cf. Ludwig et al. 2011), but it is less common, more complicated and, notably, less in the interests of private health care providers, insurance companies or drug manufacturers. As such, imposing a hierarchy of evidence, even in the field of health care, risks the introduction of issue bias if it leads to the prioritisation of treatments over prevention simply because the former are more conducive to experimental evaluation.

Discussion

There is a fundamental difference worth reiterating between using evidence for technical planning, where goals are agreed, and using evidence to inform political choices, where goals are contested. A political approach to public policy typically begins from a premise that policymaking involves choosing between competing values, objectives or social outcomes. This perspective has led Lin (2003) to describe policymaking as a situation of 'competing rationalities', with technical evidence serving as only one of the multiple concerns that must be considered in the policy process.

Advocates of EBP can of course find this perspective frustrating. The idea that evidence is only one factor in the decision-making process appears to excuse the dismissal, misuse or manipulation of scientific evidence, or it seems to imply that fidelity to science does not matter because policy makers have other concerns. This chapter, however, has aimed at clarifying the oft-muddied waters between these two sides to show that both the advocates of EBP and their critics have legitimate concerns over bias – but with two very different forms of bias in mind.

The chapter has further noted that establishing rules that impose hierarchies of evidence to direct political decisions can be a particularly important form of issue bias for the EBP movement to recognise. Imposing such rules can potentially 'mobilise bias', to use Bachrach and Baratz's (1970) term, by systematically giving priority to particular policy choices and options, such as where experimental trials or rigorous evaluations have been conducted. However, doing so privileges those groups whose interests are served by trials in particular – be they corporate actors selling treatments or population groups whose needs are more visible and more easily measured than others.

The multiple politics of evidence

These concerns work to illustrate why distinguishing between technical bias and issue bias can be particularly important. Unpacking these concepts has shown that not only are there concerns over the politics of evidence, but also that there can, in fact, be multiple politics of evidence. Technical and issue bias can arise in the creation, selection and interpretation of evidence, and Table 3.1 below presents a basic framework bringing these insights together.

Table 3.1 A multiple politics of evidence framework

	Technical bias (Politicisation of the scientific process)	*Issue bias* (Depoliticisation of the policy process)
Creation of evidence	Designing a study to advance a desired policy goal. Altering study design mid-stream to produce positive findings.	Obfuscation of the value choices or of the value implications arising from the: • choice of topic to research (e.g. HIV/tuberculosis/malaria research versus neglected tropical diseases); • availability of data or feasibility to generate evidence (e.g. marginalised or hidden populations); • selection of outcomes to include (e.g. 'harms' of injecting drugs measured as health outcomes, or the 'message' it sends about appropriate behaviour).
Selection of evidence	'Cherry-picking' and strategic review of data to justify a pre-determined position.	Presenting a policy option as 'evidence-based' while utilising evidence from a sub-set of relevant policy concerns.
Interpretation of evidence	Erroneous interpretations in policy debates, e.g. premature causal claims about a preferred strategy; confused understandings of risk.	Unwarranted interpretations of the importance of evidence, e.g. interpreting methodological rigour as an indication of policy relevance.

Delineating between these multiple politics of evidence is important for a number of reasons. First, it helps to overcome the apparent debates between champions and critics of the EBP movement by illustrating that both have valid concerns and clarifying the different normative ideals these groups embrace. The framework further helps to illustrate when and how such forms of bias may arise. This can subsequently allow us to ask much more direct questions about how political factors serve to drive different forms of bias, which can inform thinking of how to improve the use of evidence in policymaking by overcoming both forms of bias. It is to these questions that we now turn in the next two chapters.

References

Aubrey, Alison. 2015. 'Even if you're lean, 1 soda per day ups your risk of diabetes'. NPR. http://www.npr.org/sections/thesalt/2015/07/23/425635400/even-if-youre-lean-1-soda-per-day-ups-your-risk-of-diabetes?sc=tw, accessed 23 June 2016.

Bachrach, Peter and Morton Baratz. 1970. *Power and Poverty: Theory and Practice.* Oxford: Oxford University Press.

Barnes, Amy and Justin Parkhurst. 2014. 'Can global health policy be depoliticised? A critique of global calls for evidence-based policy'. In *Handbook of Global Health Policy*, edited by Gavin Yamey and Garrett Brown, pp. 157–173. Chichester: Wiley-Blackwell.

Begley, C. Glenn. 2013. 'Six red flags for suspect work'. *Nature* 497 (23 May): 433–434.

Bekelman, J. E., Y. Li and C. P. Gross. 2003. 'Scope and impact of financial conflicts of interest in biomedical research: A systematic review'. *JAMA* 289(4): 454–465. doi: 10.1001/jama.289.4.454.

Bero, Lisa A. 2005. 'Tobacco industry manipulation of research'. *Public Health Reports* 120(2): 200–208.

Bruce-Briggs, Barry. 1976. 'The great American gun war'. *The Public Interest* 45: 37–62.

Burger, James B. 2002. *Can Gun Control Work?* Oxford: Oxford University Press.

Cameron, William Bruce. 1963. *Informal Sociology: A Casual Introduction to Sociological Thinking*. New York: Random House.

Cao, Yin, Walter C. Willett, Eric B. Rimm, Meir J. Stampfer and Edward L. Giovannucci. 2015. 'Light to moderate intake of alcohol, drinking patterns, and risk of cancer: Results from two prospective US cohort studies'. *BMJ*, 351.

CBC News. 2011. 'Vancouver's Insite drug injection clinic will stay open', 30 September. http://www.cbc.ca/news/canada/british-columbia/vancouver-s-insite-drug-injection-clinic-will-stay-open-1.1005044, accessed 23 June 2016.

Cohen, David J., Ben Van Hout, Patrick W. Serruys, Friedrich W. Mohr, Carlos Macaya, Peter den Heijer, M. M. Vrakking, Kaijun Wang, Elizabeth M. Mahoney, Salma Audi, Katrin Leadley, Keith D. Dawkins and A. Pieter Kappetein. 2011. 'Quality of life after PCI with drug-eluting stents or coronary-artery bypass surgery'. *New England Journal of Medicine* 364(11): 1016–1026. doi: 10.1056/NEJMoa1001508.

Culp-Ressler, Tara. 2013. 'President Obama defends age restrictions on over-the-counter emergency contraception'. http://thinkprogress.org/health/2013/05/03/1958521/president-obama-defends-age-restrictions-plan-b.

Cummings, K. Michael, Anthony Brown and Richard O'Connor. 2007. 'The cigarette controversy'. *Cancer Epidemiology Biomarkers & Prevention* 16(6): 1070–1076. doi: 10.1158/1055-9965.epi-06-0912.

Dennis, Brady and Sarah Kliff. 2013. 'Obama administration drops fight to keep age restrictions on Plan B sales'. *Washington Post*, 10 June.

Di Nicola, Andrea. 2007. 'Researching into human trafficking: Issues and problems'. In *Human Trafficking*, edited by Maggy Lee, pp. 49–72. Cullompton: Willan Publishing.

Dobbs, David. 2015. 'The human cost of a misleading drug-safety study'. *The Atlantic*, 18 September.

Douglas, Heather. 2015. 'Politics and science: Untangling values, ideologies, and reasons'. *Annals of the American Academy of Political and Social Science* 658(1): 296–306. doi: 10.1177/0002716214557237.

Duncan, David Ewing. 2007. 'The anti-science president'. *MIT Technology Review*. http://www.technologyreview.com/view/408236/the-anti-science-president, accessed 23 June 2016. *The Economist*. 2016. 'For my next trick . . . ' *The Economist* 418(8982): 82–83.

EurActive.com. 2014. 'EU twisting facts to fit political agenda, chief scientist says'. http://www.euractiv.com/sections/eu-priorities-2020/eu-twisting-facts-fit-political-agenda-chief-scientist-says-302399, accessed 23 June 2016.

Fanelli, Daniele. 2009. 'How many scientists fabricate and falsify research? A systematic review and meta-analysis of survey data'. *PLoS ONE* 4(5): e5738. doi: 10.1371/journal.pone.0005738.

Fries, James F. and Eswar Krishnan. 2004. 'Equipoise, design bias, and randomized controlled trials: The elusive ethics of new drug development'. *Arthritis Research & Theory* 6(3): R250–R255.

Giles, Jim. 2006. 'UK civil servants accused of warping science'. *Nature* 444(7117): 252–253.

Goldacre, Ben. 2014. *Bad Pharma: How Drug Companies Mislead Doctors and Harm Patients*. London: Fourth Estate.

Gordon, Stephen, John Smyth and Julie Diehl. 2008. 'The Iraq war, "sound science", and "evidence-based" educational reform: How the Bush administration uses deception, manipulation, and subterfuge to advance its chosen ideology'. *Journal for Critical Education Policy Studies* 6(2): 173–204.

Haskins, Ron and Jon Baron. 2011. *Building the Connection between Policy and Evidence: The Obama Evidence-Based Initatives*. London: NESTA.

Hersh, Seymour M. 2003. 'The annals of security: The Stovepipe'. *The New Yorker*, 27 September. http://www.newyorker.com/magazine/2003/10/27/the-stovepipe, accessed 23 June 2016.

Hotez, Peter and Aruna Kamath. 2009. 'Neglected tropical diseases in Sub-Saharan Africa: Review of their prevalence, distribution, and disease burden'. *PLoS Neglected Tropical Diseases* 3(8): e412. doi: 10.1371/journal.pntd.0000412.

House of Commons Science and Technology Committee. 2006. *Scientific Advice, Risk and Evidence Based Policy Making*. London: The Stationery Office.

Hurt, Richard D., Jon O. Ebbert, Monique E. Muggli, Nikki J. Lockhart and Channing R. Robertson. 2009. 'Open doorway to truth: Legacy of the Minnesota tobacco trial'. *Mayo Clinic Proceedings* 84(5): 446–456.

Imamura, Fumiaki, Laura O'Connor, Zheng Ye, Jaakko Mursu, Yasuaki Hayashino, Shilpa Bhupathiraju and Nita Forouhi. 2015. 'Consumption of sugar sweetened beverages, artificially sweetened beverages, and fruit juice and incidence of type 2 diabetes: Systematic review, meta-analysis, and estimation of population attributable fraction'. *British Medical Journal* 351. doi 10.1136/bmj.h3576.

Institute of Climate Studies. 'Climate science data: Cherry picking'. http://www.icsusa.org/pages/articles/2013-icsusa-articles/may-2013---climate-science-data-cherry-picking.php#.VV971UYku4E, accessed 23 June 2016.

Jasanoff, Sheila. 1987. 'Contested boundaries in policy-relevant science'. *Social Studies of Science* 17(2): 195–230.

——. 2006. 'Biotechnology and empire: The global power of seeds and science'. *Osiris* 21(1): 273–292. doi: 10.1086/507145.

Joint Academies of Science. Undated. 'Joint science academies' statement: Global response to climate change' http://nationalacademies.org/onpi/06072005.pdf.

Kirby, D. 2008. 'Changes in sexual behaviour leading to the decline in the prevalence of HIV in Uganda: Confirmation from multiple sources of evidence'. *Sexually Transmitted Infections* 84(Suppliment II): i35–i41.

Kleck, Gary. 1986. 'Policy lessons from recent gun control research'. *Law and Contemporary Problems* 49(1): 35–62.

Krieger, Nancy. 1992. 'The making of public health data: Paradigms, politics, and policy'. *Journal of Public Health Policy* 13: 412–427.

Le Noury, Joanna, John Nardo, David Healy, Jon Jureidini, Melissa Raven, Catalin Tufanaru and Elia Abi-Jaoude. 2015. 'Restoring study 329: Efficacy and harms of paroxetine and imipramine in treatment of major depression in adolescence'. *British Medical Journal* 351. doi: 10.1136/bmj.h4320.

Leenaars, Antoon and David Lester. 1997. 'The effects of gun control on the accidental death rate from firearms in Canada'. *Journal of Safety Research* 28(3): 119–122.

Lin, Vivian. 2003. 'Competing rationalities: evidence-based health policy'. In *Evidence-Based Health Policy: Problems & Possibilities*, edited by Vivian Lin and Brendan Gibson, pp. 3–17. Oxford: Oxford University Press.

Ludwig, Jens, Lisa Sanbonmatsu, Lisa Gennetian, Emma Adam, Greg J. Duncan, Lawrence F. Katz, Ronald C. Kessler, Jeffrey R. Kling, Stacy Tessler Lindau, Robert C. Whitaker and Thomas W. McDade. 2011. 'Neighborhoods, obesity, and diabetes – a randomized social experiment'. *New England Journal of Medicine* 365(16): 1509–1519. doi: 10.1056/NEJMsa1103216.

Lundh, Andreas, Sergio Sismondo, Joel Lexchin, Octavian A. Busuioc and Lisa Bero. 2012. 'Industry sponsorship and research outcome'. *Cochrane Database of Systematic Reviews* 12. doi 10.1002/14651858.MR000033.pub2.

MacQueen, Ken and Martin Patriquin. 2011. 'Are we ready to subsidize heroin?' http://www.macleans.ca/news/canada/are-we-ready-to-subsidize-heroin, accessed 23 June 2016.

Mooney, Chris. 2006. *The Republican War on Science.* New York: Basic Books.

Ottawa Citizen. 2006. 'Tories scrap AIDS policy statement', 18 August.

Parkhurst, Justin. 2002. 'The Ugandan success story? Evidence and claims of HIV-1 prevention'. *The Lancet* 360 (6 July): 78–80.

——. 2013. 'The subtle politics of AIDS: Values, bias, and persistent errors in HIV prevention'. In *Global HIV/AIDS Politics, Policy, and Activism*, edited by Raymond A. Smith, pp. 113–139. Santa Barbara, CA: Praeger.

Pigliucci, Massimo. 2002. *Denying Evolution: Creationism, Scientism, and the Nature of Science*. Sunderland, MA: Sinauer Associates.

Pillar, Paul R. 2006. 'Intelligence, policy, and the war in Iraq'. *Foreign Affairs*, March/April.

Piot, Peter, Coll Seck and Awa Marie. 2001. 'International response to the HIV/AIDS epidemic: Planning for success'. *Bulletin of the World Health Organization* 79(12): 1106–1112.

Putzel, James. 2004. Governance and AIDS in Africa: Assessing the international community's 'multisectoral approach'. Paper read at the Annual Meeting of the American Political Science Association, 2–5 September, Chicago.

Rampton, S. and J. Stauber. 2001. *Trust Us, We're Experts: How Industry Manipulates Science and Gambles with Your Future*. New York: Putnam.

Remme, Jan H. F., Erik Blas, Lester Chitsulo, Philippe M. P. Desjeux, Howard D. Engers, Thomas P. Kanyok, Jane F. Kengeya Kayondo, Deborah W. Kioy, Vasanthapuram Kumaraswami, Janis K. Lazdins, Paul P. Nunn, Ayoade Oduola, Robert G. Ridley, Yeya T. Toure, Fabio Zicker and Carlos M. Morel. 2002. 'Strategic emphases for tropical diseases research: A TDR perspective'. *Trends in Parasitology* 18(10):421–426. doi: http://dx.doi.org/10.1016/S1471-4922(02)02387-5.

Roberts, Michelle. 'Cancer risk "even from light drinking"'. *BBC News*, 19 August. http://www.bbc.co.uk/news/health-33975946, accessed 23 June 2016.

Russell, Jill, Trisha Greenhalgh, Emma Byrne and Janet McDonnell. 2008. 'Recognizing rhetoric in health care policy analysis'. *Journal of Health Services Research & Policy* 13(1): 40–46. doi: 10.1258/jhsrp.2007.006029.

Southwick, Lawrence. 2000. 'Self-defense with guns: The consequences'. *Journal of Criminal Justice* 28(5): 351–370.

Tong, Elisa K. and Stanton A. Glantz. 2007. 'Tobacco industry efforts undermining evidence linking secondhand smoke with cardiovascular disease'. *Circulation* 116(16): 1845–1854. doi: 10.1161/circulationaha.107.715888.

Tyldum, Guri and Anette Brunovskis. 2005. 'Describing the unobserved: Methodological challenges in empirical studies on human trafficking'. *International Migration* 43(1/2): 17–34.

UNAIDS. 1999. *Acting Early to Prevent AIDS: The Case of Senegal*. Geneva: UNAIDS.

——. 2012. *Senegal: A Success Story of AIDS Investments and Impact*. http://www.unaids.org/en/resources/presscentre/featurestories/2012/october/20121011senegal, accessed 23 June 2016.

UNAIDS and Wellcome Trust. 1999. *Trends in HIV Incidence and Prevalence: Natural Course of the Epidemic or Results of Behaviour Change?* Geneva: UNAIDS.

Union of Concerned Scientists. 2004. *Scientific Integrity in Policymaking: An Investigation into the Bush Administration's Misuse of Science*. Cambridge, MA: Union of Concerned Scientists.

Van der Heide, Liesbeth. 2013. 'Cherry-picked intelligence. The weapons of mass destruction dispositive as a legitimation for national security in the post-9/11 age'. *Historical Social Research/Historische Sozialforschung* 286–307.

Vigen, Tyler. 2015. *Spurious Correlations*. New York: Hachette Books.

Weiss, Carol H. 1979. 'The many meanings of research utilization'. *Public Administration Review* 39(5): 426–431.

——. 1998. 'Have we learned anything new about the use of evaluation?' *American Journal of Evaluation* 19(1): 21–33.

White House. 2009. 'President Barack Obama's inaugural address'. http://www.whitehouse.gov/node/1740, accessed 23 June 2016.

Wertz, Marcia, Thomas Kyriss, Suman Paranjape and Stanton Glantz. 2011. 'The toxic effects of cigarette additives. Philip Morris' project mix reconsidered: An analysis of documents released through litigation'. *PLoS Medicine* 8(12): e1001145.

White House Office of the Press Secretary. 2013. 'Press briefing by Press Secretary Jay Carney, 4/5/2013'. https://www.whitehouse.gov/the-press-office/2013/04/05/press-briefing-press-secretary-jay-carney-452013, accessed 23 June 2016.

Whitehouse, David. 2014. 'The cherry-picking climate change committee'. Global Warming Policy Forum. http://www.thegwpf.com/cherry-picking-climate-committee, accessed 23 June 2016.

Wood, Evan, Mark Tyndall, Julio Montaner and Thomas Kerr. 2006. 'Summary of findings from the evaluation of a pilot medically supervised safer injecting facility'. *Canadian Medical Association Journal* 175(11): 1399–1404.

4 The overt politics of evidence

Bias and the pursuit of political interests

Politics as competition and contestation

As has already been discussed, a common critique of the EBP movement is how many discussions under this heading seem to address evidence use without any direct engagement with the concept of politics. This is despite numerous authors explaining that the nature of policymaking is inherently political, and the role of evidence in such cases will therefore be fundamentally different to instances of technical problem solving (cf. Cartwright and Hardie 2012; Davies, Nutley and Smith 2000; Greenhalgh and Russell 2009; Nutley, Walter and Davies 2007; Parsons 2002; Weiss 1991). This chapter, however, presents the first of two explorations into how the political nature of policymaking may result in different forms of technical and issue bias. Specifically, it describes instances of bias that arise from the pursuit of political interests within a contested and competitive political environment.

For academics within the field of public policy (and political science more broadly), the fact that policy decisions are contested is not only recognised, but can also be a principal reason to study policymaking in the first place. Many date the origins of the modern field of public policy, for example, to the work of Harold Lasswell (cf. DeLeon 2006), who has been described as the father of a 'policy sciences' movement that aimed to develop scientifically informed efforts to provide political solutions to social needs (Lasswell 1971; Lerner and Lasswell 1951). This is a decidedly goal-oriented approach, but even so, Lasswell recognised that the process by which those social needs were determined would involve trade-offs between interest groups (Lasswell 1990 [1936]). David Easton, writing in the 1950s, similarly noted that: '[The] essence of a policy lies in the fact that through it certain things are denied to some people and made accessible to others. A policy . . . consists of a web of decisions and actions that allocates values' (1971 [1953], pp. 129–130). In more recent years, Heywood has explained that: 'Politics is . . . inextricably linked to the phenomena of *conflict* and *cooperation* . . . the existence of rival opinions, different wants, competing needs and opposing interests guarantees disagreement about the rules under which people live' (2007, p. 2, emphasis in original).

From a public policy perspective, then, what makes something *political* is the existence of disagreement over values and competition between groups.

The seemingly ubiquitous phenomena of policy advocacy and lobbying illustrates this point. These are typically understood as representing organised efforts to shift governmental policies to the desired outcomes of particular interest groups (cf. Baumgartner and Leech 1998; Baumgartner et al. 2009). The policy process thus serves as an arena of competition in many cases. This recognition is also reflected in contemporary conceptual frameworks that aim to describe processes of policy change. One of the most widely applied of these is that of the Advocacy Coalitions Framework, which describes policy change as occurring through an ongoing and continuous process of competition between separate coalitions who differ in their sets of policy-relevant beliefs (Sabatier 1988, 2007).

Seeing policymaking as defined by competition over interests and beliefs, and conceptualising the policy process as the arena through which that competition occurs, has fundamental implications for our understanding of the politics of evidence, however. In particular, it becomes much more obvious that participation in policy debates is not driven by a desire to be technically accurate, but rather by a need for political success or even survival. And it is this reality that can provide the first pillar on which to explore when, why and how technical and issue bias can manifest themselves in political processes. These manifestations are described here as representing an *overt* politics of evidence, not necessarily because every instance of bias is easily recognised, but as they derive from deliberate strategies taken in the pursuit of political interests (in the next chapter we examine a second way in which politics can engender bias that may be less deliberate and, as such, much more *subtle*).

Interests and technical bias

Achieving a desired policy decision

One of the most basic ways in which political interests can drive technical bias is when groups strategically manipulate evidence in order to increase the chance that a policy decision results in a favoured outcome. Examples provided in the previous chapter illustrated a number of cases where corporate actors used evidence in such ways in order to result in a favourable decision being made about their product (whether it is to promote use of a drug or to avoid regulation or restriction of a product). The reasons why this happens, of course, are not hard to understand. Businesses are not typically driven by a motivation for scientific accuracy or good evidentiary practice; rather, businesses pursue profit.

It is often said that not only do businesses pursue profit, but they are also legally mandated to maximise shareholder value. Whether this is true or not may depend on the laws of particular countries (and, indeed, how those laws are interpreted; cf. Stout 2008). Yet even if there is no official legal requirement for corporate profit maximisation, basic economic theory tells us that in perfectly competitive markets with free entry and exit, any firm not maximising profit risks being supplanted by another that will. However, taking the profit motive as the principal goal of corporations makes their political strategies with regard to evidence much more predictable.

As in the previous chapter, we can again look at the tobacco industry for easy-to-find examples. In 2013, for instance, the UK government was considering passing legislation that would remove branding from cigarette packages – requiring so-called 'standardised packaging' (or 'plain packaging') which had been piloted previously in Australia as a smoking reduction measure. One large tobacco company, Japan Tobacco International (JTI), which opposed this measure, went so far as to place full-page advertisements in British newspapers claiming that the proposal was not 'evidence-based policy', but rather 'policy-based evidence' (although the adverts were subsequently banned by advertising regulators for making false claims, Thomas 2013).[1] Nevertheless, the irony of the tobacco industry making such claims can quickly be seen when considering the results of academic investigations of the industry's tactics. Ulucanlar et al. (2014), for instance, found a number of problematic aspects of the tobacco industry's use of evidence to argue against standardised packaging, including insisting on unrealistic methodological perfection of evaluations, misquoting published studies and withholding evidence, in order to push their case in the UK.

Yet we can ask if we should be surprised by such findings. Tobacco companies are clearly taking the role of an interest group and, indeed, how this affects their use of evidence has been explained by Bero (2005) after investigating tobacco company manipulation of research. She states that 'an interest group is an organized group with a narrowly defined viewpoint, which protects its position or profits . . . Interest groups *can be expected* to construct the evidence about a health risk to support their predefined policy position' (2005, p. 200, emphasis added). She then lists the following set of strategies the tobacco industry has particularly utilised to do this:

> 1 Fund research that supports the interest group position.
> 2 Publish research that supports the interest group position.
> 3 Suppress research that does not support the interest group position.
> 4 Criticize research that does not support the interest group position.
> 5 Disseminate interest group data or interpretation of risk in the lay press.
> 6 Disseminate interest group data or interpretation of risk directly to policy makers.
>
> (2005, p. 200)

One of Bero's points is that we should *expect* the strategic use of evidence by interest groups pursuing policy positions rather than seeing it as an aberration or somehow surprising. However, this expectation arises from the understanding that policymaking is characterised by competition. In a competitive environment,

1 As of April 2016, pdfs of the adverts can be found at: http://www.jti.com/files/4313/4910/2125/JTI_Ads_July.pdf.

lobbyists would be acting 'rationally' to use whatever evidence they can (and in whatever way they can) to achieve the desired outcome. As such, the competitive nature of policy decision making provides the incentive structure driving technical bias in key ways.

And it is not only corporate actors pursuing financial interests that this affects. The field of political advocacy reaches well beyond financial interests, yet is similarly driven by a desire to achieve preferred goals and social outcomes. Perfectly selfless individuals working in areas of policy advocacy can similarly face situations where pieces of evidence conflict with a desired outcome, thereby producing pressure towards bias. In these cases, a conflict of interest exists – not a financial conflict per se, but one that still can result in pieces of evidence being used strategically to pursue desired political goals. Indeed, writing in the journal *Nature*, Pielke argues that: 'Political advocates will always selectively use and misuse scientific data to support their agendas' (2002, p. 368), giving examples of climate change, nuclear power and biodiversity as particularly illustrative cases in point.

Pressure to show results

An alternative way in which the competitive nature of policymaking can engender bias arises not just from individuals attempting to achieve a policy decision in their favour, but also when those already in positions of authority use evidence in biased ways to demonstrate positive programme results or, alternatively, to hide unwanted findings. The pressure to do so can again arise from the competitive nature of the political system, but in this case it can be competition for officials to maintain their position, status or support from those to whom they are held accountable. So elected officials will be under pressure to gain votes to be re-elected; politically appointed bureaucrats need to be successful in order to keep their jobs; and heads of social programmes are regularly asked to show evidence of success in order to justify and maintain their budgets in the face of competing demands for resources. However, such pressures can obviously create incentives for biased uses of evidence, and it is not difficult to find cases where public officials in positions of authority have been accused of manipulating evidence to show better results.

In 2015, for example, the *New York Times* reported that: 'The Pentagon's inspector general is investigating allegations that military officials have skewed intelligence assessments about the United States-led campaign in Iraq against the Islamic State to provide a more optimistic account of progress' (Mazzetti and Apuzzoaug 2015). In the US there have been a fair number of accusations of evidence manipulation in the education sector as well. Recent media attention, for instance, focused on the court conviction and sentencing of 11 educators in the city of Atlanta on felony charges for altering student standardised test results (Blinder 2015) – and this was just one of a range of 'cheating scandals' in recent years. In other cases, teachers were found directly changing students' exam answers or excluding poor-performing students from tests to improve results (cf. Beckett 2013; Vogell 2011). The frequency of educator 'cheating' by manipulating evidence of student performance has even been estimated by Jacob and Levitt for the city of Chicago. Their analysis concluded that 'serious cases of teacher or administrator cheating on standardized tests occur in a minimum of 4–5 percent of elementary school classrooms annually' (Jacob and Levitt 2003, p. 843).

The pressure to show results can drive evidentiary bias in international public agencies as well. Hickel, for instance, has described how an agency of the United Nations appears to have changed the metrics by which it measures the number of hungry people in the world in order to look more successful in the achievement of the Millennium Development Goals (MDGs – a set of globally agreed development goals to be reached by 2015). He explains that up until 2012, data were showing a trend of increasing global hunger rates, but:

> at the end of 2012, the news changed. With only three years to go before the expiry of the MDGs, the UN's Food and Agricultural Organisation (FAO) announced an 'improved' methodology for counting hunger. And the revised numbers delivered a rosy tale at last: while 23% of the developing world was undernourished in 1990, the UN was pleased to announce a reduction down to 15%. The goal still wasn't in reach, but at least the millennium campaign could finally claim some progress.
>
> (Hickel 2015; see also Hickel 2016)

Such examples – manipulating evidence on a war's progress, on children's educational outcomes or on the number of hungry people in the world – may seem particularly egregious, and it may seem surprising to consider these were done by public servants, not corporate actors. But it is important to understand how such bias can arise if there is a desire to prevent it in the future. The nature of competition within policy sectors naturally incentivises bias in cases such as these. Indeed, Stephen Levitt, co-author of the Chicago cheating study (as well as the popular book *Freakonomics*), has argued that the rewards placed on doing well in standardised testing naturally produces incentives to manipulate evidence, explaining: 'The way teachers respond to incentives is just human nature . . . To quote W. C. Fields: "Anything worth winning is worth cheating for"' (Levitt 2005).

Finally, a slightly different manifestation of the pressure to show results can also arise when evidence is hidden or not released because it is politically sensitive. Examples seen in 2015 alone include: the Indian government being accused of failing to release health survey data results, presumably because it showed particularly poor results in Gujerat (where the Prime Minister previously served as State Chief Minister) (*BBC News* 2015); the UK government being accused of failing to release data on the number of people who have died within six weeks of having their government benefits stopped (Brown 2015); and the Chinese government being accused of hiding urban pollution data from the public to protect polluting industries (Chen 2015). Again, each of these cases can be seen as a case of technical bias that has arisen from a competitive political environment in which support, or even political survival, may be undermined by a robust or systematic provision of evidence.

Undermining science as a political strategy

While there may be an abundance of cases of governments, corporations or interest groups hiding or manipulating individual data, there can also be cases where political interests are so challenged by bodies of evidence that affected stakeholders decide to pursue a strategy to undermine the whole of the scientific exercise. Chapter 1 gave as an example the accusations levelled against the Exxon corporation that it supported groups challenging scientific consensus after early research showed the potential harms of climate change (Hall 2015). In their recent book *Merchants of Doubt*, Oreskes and Conway (2011) explore further how organised corporate interests construct doubt, manipulate the scientific process or undermine the credibility of research processes to advance political goals for issues such as tobacco, ozone depletion, acid rain and strategic defence.

One particularly common strategy in these efforts has been to make calls for scientific 'proof' before political action can take place. This can particularly be seen in climate change debates, although it also arises at other times – such as in debates over teaching evolution in schools when proponents of creationism criticise evolution as 'only a theory'. Yet 'proof' is typically not what science provides and is not the point of appealing to evidence. Oreskes (2004) explains: 'In all but the most trivial cases, science does not produce logically indisputable proofs about the natural world. At best it produces a robust consensus based on a process of inquiry that allows for continued scrutiny, re-examination, and revision' (2004, p. 369).

Undermining aspects of the scientific exercise might appear to some as a short-sighted means to political ends. Yet when the survival – financial or ideological – of an interest group is at stake, it may be a perfectly 'rational' strategy to try to undermine the power or influence of scientific evidence in policy deliberations. The tobacco industry's products are known to be harmful and, as such, any scientific research on the harms of smoking or, alternatively, on the effectiveness of smoking cessation interventions will have negative impacts on the industry's future economic survival. Thus, it is quite reasonable to consider whether creating a culture of doubt or scepticism over science would better serve the industry's goals than embracing evidentiary best practice.

Again, however, it is not just corporate actors who may do this. There are, of course, historical cases where religious authorities have challenged the scientific establishment as well (Russell 1997). Religious institutions have served as dominant centres of power for millennia, and their legitimacy has, in many ways, relied on being seen as an accurate authority on how the world (and the heavens above) functions. Historians of science and religion now reject the widely held 'conflict thesis', which argues that religion and science are fundamentally irreconcilable (Brooke 1991) – yet there are clearly cases where scientific findings have proved threatening to institutionalised theological centres of power. So whether it is observations of the phases of Venus indicating that planets orbit the sun, radiometric dating indicating that the earth is billions of years old or fossil analyses illustrating the evolution of hominids, there will be some who will see these outcomes of scientific enquiry as an existential threat, providing a strong incentive to challenge scientific practice itself.

Interests and issue bias

The pursuit of competing interests within the political arena can also drive examples of issue bias, whereby the creation, selection and use of evidence directs policy attention to a limited number of key concerns and acts to obscure other relevant policy considerations. Indeed, while lobbyists and advocates may face pressure to manipulate or hide evidence at times, as discussed above, a great deal of advocacy is primarily aimed at increasing the weight or priority that decision makers give to their interests, or to convince policy makers that their concerns are the most relevant for policy action. Simply pursuing an interest or promoting one set of values over another is not necessarily issue bias, however; rather, the term more specifically reflects cases when political prioritisation is obscured by the language and rules of evidence utilisation.

The previous chapter identified issue bias in a number of contemporary policy issues. The example of gun control in the US was one such case demonstrating that there can be many social concerns at stake in political debate and, as such, many bodies of potentially relevant evidence to draw upon. It is unsurprising, then, that gun control advocates routinely point to evidence speaking to their core concerns over individual and societal harms, such as research showing relationships between gun ownership and homicide or suicide deaths (cf. Fleegler et al. 2013). However, gun control opponents typically espouse the values of personal choice or freedom, and it is equally unsurprising that they instead point to evidence speaking to these interests, such as surveys that indicate a general public opposition to the idea of banning guns (cf. Jones 2011). Both sides use their preferred evidence to try to influence policy decisions and both may claim to therefore be pursuing an 'evidence-based policy' in their opposite policy positions.

It is from this perspective that critics of the EBP movement raise concerns about how the promotion of evidence can, at times, *depoliticise* the policymaking process. This is because there is a strong assumption at times that evidence is somehow *apolitical*, and the terminology of 'evidence-based policy' has a clear implication that there must be a single *correct* policy choice that the evidence legitimates or justifies. Yet, as the gun control example shows, opposing coalitions may both present 'evidence-based' policies. Issue bias arises when this fundamentally normative debate over social values becomes confused as an evaluation of evidence – allowing political interests to be introduced through what Wesselink and colleagues (2014) described as the 'back door' – hiding debates over values within the language of evidence utilisation. Values and evidence may both be important to decision making and there is a clear need not to get them confused in such cases.

Selective knowledge transfer and evidence-based advocacy

However, the recognition that pieces of evidence can reflect particular interests raises questions about many of the common knowledge transfer efforts in which specific pieces of evidence are promoted for 'uptake' into policy and practice. While there are some authors who have reflected more broadly on systems or structures in place to provide evidence to decision makers (cf. Chew, Armstrong and Martin 2013; Lavis et al. 2013; Ongolo-Zogo et al. 2014), a large proportion of the knowledge transfer literature has been concerned instead with trying to identify ways to get specific pieces of research evidence 'used' by decision makers (Langer, Tripney and Gough 2016). This approach typically embraces efforts of knowledge brokering as a way to get past the 'messiness' of political decision making (cf. Ward, House and Hamer 2009), with knowledge brokers or intermediaries seen as conduits through which policy 'impact' can be achieved for specific pieces of research (cf. Chew, Armstrong and Martin 2013, Dobbins et al. 2009, van Kammen, de Savigny and Sewankambo 2006). Yet once knowledge brokering shifts from a service that informs *multiple* potential considerations, or that provides evidence on request for a representative authority, to one of a strategy to *achieve change* by getting specific pieces of research 'into' policy, it can become an advocacy strategy in all but name.

Most discussion in the knowledge transfer literature fails to recognise that the decision over which evidence to promote will be a political choice (Liverani, Hawkins and Parkhurst 2013; Smith 2013). Rather, such work often rests on the widely critiqued assumption that evidence use is inherently an uncontested 'good thing', with 'politics' seen to be a negative 'barrier' to research utilisation – a barrier that needs to be overcome (cf. Oliver et al. 2014; Oliver, Lorenc and Innvaer 2014, Rutter, Hawkins and Parkhurst 2013). However, starting instead from an understanding that policy decisions are characterised by competition over values and interests alternatively sees politics as the mechanism by which political priorities are set. Politics, from this perspective, is not something to overcome, but rather something that enables appropriate consideration to be given to relevant social concerns.

Yet, at times, evidence is explicitly used as a tool for the promotion of political interests. Mably (2006), for instance, uses the term 'evidence-based advocacy' to refer to the work done by international non-government organisations (NGOs) in providing research to influence policy in line with their agendas in the field of international trade. The United Nations Children's Emergency Fund (UNICEF) has similarly produced an 'advocacy toolkit' in which one strategy promoted is to generate 'evidence for advocacy' so as to influence decisions in line with their interests in 'improving children's lives' (UNICEF 2010). The World Health Organization (WHO 2012) has also used the term 'evidence-based advocacy' to explain how analyses of local country level data can be developed into advocacy materials to 'build stakeholder commitment' for policy actions to improve reproductive, maternal and newborn health. The UNICEF toolkit report explicitly justifies its approach by referring to its mandate from the UN General Assembly to advocate for children's rights, needs and opportunities, while the WHO's strategic use of evidence is more implicitly justified in terms of achieving progress towards the Millennium Development Goals. But in both cases, the organisations are promoting the use of issue-specific evidence to shape national government policy decisions towards preferred interests. Even though many readers may see goals such as improving maternal or child health as laudable, it is important to recognise that if there is a need to raise the priority of the issue or to build commitment in the first place, there are likely to be other competing interests or concerns at stake in the political decision-making process (whether socially desirable or not) that, in these cases, the use of evidence is strategically aimed to defeat.

Appeals to evidence as a rhetorical strategy

It is also increasingly common to see strategic appeals to evidence serving as a rhetorical device in order to make a particular interest group appear more legitimate. In UNICEF's advocacy toolkit, for example, the organisation states: 'Evidence for advocacy provides credibility and authority to the organization, allowing us to convince decision makers to support an issue' (UNICEF 2010, p. 11). The credibility that comes from embracing scientific evidence, then, is seen to be useful to convince policymakers as much as any argument about the need to improve children's rights and social outcomes in and of themselves. However, a contrasting example can be seen in the case discussed earlier of the tobacco company JTI claiming that UK government proposals on standardised packaging, labelling an unwanted proposal as 'not evidence-based' to try to diminish its perceived legitimacy.

These examples show just how strategic and malleable the term 'evidence-based policy' can be when used in policy debates. In the JTI case, the corporation used this language to resist a smoking reduction strategy based on plain packaging, claiming that such an intervention did not have a strong evidence base about whether it would reduce smoking rates. Yet, given the abundant evidence of the health harms of tobacco smoking, many would equally claim an 'evidence-based tobacco policy' could be to ban it outright or perhaps to instigate any and all restrictive measures possible. Authors like Myers (2013) have used language in this way to discuss the use of 'evidence-based policies' to achieve a tobacco 'end-game' that eliminates the tobacco epidemic completely.

Clearly there is no single or indisputable answer to what an 'evidence-based tobacco policy' actually is or what the final goals should be. There is an abundance of evidence about the health harms of smoking. There are various pieces of evidence about the efficacy of different intervention strategies that might reduce smoking. And there are other pieces of evidence speaking to concerns about the social acceptability of smoking, the importance of personal freedom to population groups, or the economic benefits or costs of smoking to different sectors of society (from tax revenue to retail sales to health expenditure). Any piece of this agglomeration of evidence might be selected on which to 'base' a policy (or base opposition to a policy), and in competitive policy environments, there can be a range of rhetorical uses of 'evidence' that serve to frame the debate so as to include or exclude particular social concerns (Bacchi 2009; Fischer 2003; Schön and Rein 1994).

Recognition of the rhetorical nature of policy debates can therefore help us to understand how the language of 'scientific evidence' proves useful in and of itself. Science is recognised as having particular authority in policy debates due to its perception as objective and its ability to accurately represent the world (Jasanoff 1987), with Freedman (2006) describing a 'fetishizing' of scientific data within the media to reflect the authority that arises from appeals to data. This privilege given to research evidence makes it a particularly useful rhetorical strategy to invoke and has led to authors such as Hammersley to argue that calling something 'evidence-based' now serves as nothing more than a slogan used to 'discredit opposition' (2013, p. 15). While this may not always be the case, and many evidence advocates would respond by pointing back to the need to ensure that scientific best practices are followed to achieve social goals, there is clearly an important recognition to be made about how discursive use of the language of evidence can frame issues in ways that construct particular interests or ideas into, or out of, policy debates.

Expecting instances of bias

The principal goal of this chapter has been to illustrate that the fundamentally political nature of policymaking, which involves competition between different sets of beliefs or interests, provides incentives that can generate both technical bias and issue bias alike. This is because in political arenas, interest groups will compete for policy attention, and those in positions of power will compete for public support (or resources), with significant implications if they fail to achieve their goals. In such a system, there is no reason to assume that fidelity to science or accurate presentations of evidence will be a primary value amongst groups in political competition and, as such, unless these things are somehow required to obtain political or public support, they will inevitably be sacrificed when doing so can help in winning (or surviving) political competitions.

However, understanding this means that many forms of bias are likely to be *predictable* or at least can be *expected* when the political stakes are high enough. The pressure to show results (or to hide negative results) also captures what in more popular language might be referred to as political 'spin'. Yet spin (applied to evidence) can take two forms. It can involve the manipulation of evidence to show better results (or minimise problematic ones) – effectively representing technical bias – or it can involve selecting and focusing on technically valid pieces of evidence that only highlight those issues or outcomes where the political actor is doing well – effectively representing issue bias. What is key to recognise is that spin should be expected as a natural result of a highly incentivised and competitive political system.

Returning to Weiss' (1979) description of the various ways in which research can influence policy (detailed in Chapter 2), we can assume that her conceptualisation of *strategic* uses of evidence would in fact be a norm rather than an exception in many such environments. Weiss herself, for instance, has stated:

> Politicians and officials have ideological convictions and constellations of interests that largely set the course they steer. The place of information generally, and of research information particularly, is best seen as helping

> policy makers decide which policies are best suited to the realization of their ideologies and interests.
>
> (1991, p. 308)

Hoppe similarly draws on Weiss to explain that an 'adversarial' model of policy-making makes it evident when we might see strategic uses of scientific expertise. He explains that:

> Politics is the non-violent power struggle between political parties and/or organized interest groups . . . The struggle between group interests functions as variety generator and selection environment for scientific arguments that underpin political positions and decisions. Every interest involved will look for the type of scientific expertise that harnesses and legitimizes its pre-formed political stance.
>
> (Hoppe 2005, p. 210)

Evidence champions have long bemoaned the manipulation of evidence in ways that are not scientifically valid, but clearly a more nuanced understanding of political debate is required to also explore concepts of issue bias that can occur through rhetorical framing. Political rhetoric, argumentation, discourse and framing are particularly the subjects of the sub-field of critical policy studies, which explores how policy power is structured or exercised through the construction of ideas and meaning (cf. Fischer and Forrester 1993; Stone 2002; Susskind 2006). From this perspective, for instance, Bacchi (2009) argues that we are 'governed by problematisations' rather than by problems, by which she means that those things that are considered to be 'policy needs' are, in fact, constructed by how issues are represented. As such, she particularly takes issue with the EBP movement for obscuring the process by which the issues are constructed, which assigns value and fixes the concerns taken to be relevant to the policy problem. She explains:

> in evidence-based policy, objective 'problems' *are* presumed to exist, separate from power and contestation, waiting only upon 'evidence' about 'what works'. So long as 'problems' are considered to sit outside the political process (exogenous) in this way, waiting to be 'solved' through 'relevant' 'evidence', the necessarily political contestation around competing representation of 'problems' is displaced and hence ignored.
>
> (Bacchi 2009, p. 253, emphasis in original)

This reiterates the concerns raised in previous chapters over how certain uses of evidence can depoliticise the policymaking process. Not only do we need to be aware of how the language of EBP may obscure the nature of political debate, we also need to be aware of how pieces of technical evidence can be used strategically to frame the terms of the debate itself. Within policy argumentation, evidence can get used in ways that can shape just what policies are 'represented to be' (to use Bacchi's language) so as to legitimate particular policy choices and to exclude competing interests.

Understanding the problem to consider solutions

Identifying so many forms of evidentiary bias and conceptualising the political nature of policymaking as inherently driven by competition may, to some, appear to support a conclusion that bias is inevitable within policy debates. Yet understanding the origins and manifestations of bias makes instances of bias more understandable and, indeed, even predictable. This in turn permits consideration of whether particular types of policy debates may be more susceptible to bias emerging and further enables reflection on where to target strategies to reduce or mitigate the bias that is expected to arise. In particular, here we note three features of policy problems that appear relevant to engender bias: the complexity of the problem, the level of contestation (or importance) and the polarisation of the issue.

Problem complexity

Obviously many of the policy problems that rely on evidence can be described as complex. Yet 'complexity' is a broad term which can capture multiple features that can manifest in different sources of bias. One useful distinction of the concept comes from the field of complexity theory, which distinguishes between what are termed *complicated* as opposed to *complex* problems (Snowden and Boone 2007; Snyder 2013).[2] *Complicated* problems, in this distinction, are said to include multiple interacting or mutually interdependent elements, each one of which may be solvable or knowable. The stereotypical example is sending a rocket to the moon (cf. Glouberman and Zimmerman 2002): rocket science may be difficult, and getting a rocket to the moon requires multiple pieces of expertise, but the process is essentially predictable and repeatable in most cases. *Complex* issues, on the other hand, are seen to contain elements of *uncertainty* in terms of cause–effect relationships, many of which can only be identified after the fact. This can make the prediction of outcomes difficult or can lead to different outcomes if the same actions are taken in subsequent iterations (even with 'perfect' evidence available). Raising a child is often given as an example of this, but many policies and interventions designed to bring about social change in context-specific settings would also fall under this category (Glouberman and Zimmerman 2002; Kurtz and Snowden 2003).

Complicated problems are typically multifaceted, which can be seen as increasing the opportunity for issue bias, as multiple interests are likely to be

2 There are further ways to explore complexity as well. Snowden and Boone (2007), for example, delineate between simple, complicated, complex and chaotic contexts, adding two additional considerations (in chaotic cases, for example, rapid response is said to be needed in ways that eliminate the ability to even consider a rational or comprehensive assessment of evidence). We have limited the number of features of complexity to two here, as these capture the principal political mechanisms of bias that are explored here and in the next chapter.

relevant to the policy debates. Issue framing will also likely be important in complicated problems and can lead to some bodies of evidence being seen as relevant to the exclusion of others. The previous example of gun control can be considered particularly complicated given that gun restrictions may affect a range of social concerns, including accidental deaths, citizen resistance to armed criminals, tax revenues from gun sales and a host of other outcomes. Some of these have been estimated or measured in individual cases, but they each may speak to a different interest or social value.

However, in *complex* situations, the uncertainty involved provides opportunities for different forms of evidentiary bias. The sowing of doubt as a political strategy to undermine scientific credibility, for example, would likely be more effective for a complex policy issue with a number of scientific unknowns. Climate science may be a particular extreme case, where there are a huge number of variables that lead to specific outcomes at a given place and time. This might compare with different social policy debates, such as those over abortion or homosexual rights, which are highly contested but where there are significantly fewer scientific unknowns.

Contestation/importance of the issue

The level of contestation – reflected in the importance of the policy decision to the stakeholders involved – provides a second feature of policy that can influence the mechanisms through which bias arises. Some policy decisions will simply not be that highly contested and we would hardly expect to see evidence manipulation as a political strategy for fairly mundane decisions such as what day a municipality should collect recycling, or whether fire engines should be painted yellow or red. In these cases, the interests involved would not be strong enough to justify sacrificing scientific credibility to gain political advantage. Yet clearly the more important a policy decision is to interest groups, the stronger the incentive will be to manipulate evidence in pursuit of key goals – whether it is a policy affecting the profits of a corporation, the likelihood of re-election or simply the progress achieved towards a desired social objective.

Problem polarisation

A final feature of policy problems that may drive instances of bias can be the polarisation of the issue, reflecting how many policy choices are available to balance the multiple interests at stake. At one extreme would be policy decisions that can choose from a large number of intermediary positions – for instance, decisions over what teacher–student ratio to use in classrooms or how much a government should regulate free markets. A large number of options exist in these cases, and while there may be some extreme opinions on market regulation, for instance, most people would fall along a spectrum of middle-ground positions about when markets should be regulated to ensure public safety or address market failures. Highly polarised issues, on the other hand, have few middle-ground positions. Abortion or gay marriage, for instance, are typically debated over a single binary division. It is conceivable that highly polarised policy issues such as these could involve greater incentives for evidence manipulation, as the implication of an unfavourable policy decision would be extreme for the losing side of the debate. Decisions over the validity of creationism (which play out in policies regarding science curricula in schools) provide one example of a polarised issue that has little scope for compromise – either it is valid to teach creationism as science or it is not. In such cases, polarised policy debates may be seen as a 'winner take all' scenario, increasing the incentive to create or use evidence in biased ways.

Alternative conceptualisations

The choice of three policy features – complexity, contestation and polarisation – is, of course, only one way to identify potentially important aspects of policy problems. But this classification was chosen because it can be directly applied to think about the political origins of bias (as shown above and as will be further explored in the next chapter). However, other potentially useful classification systems are worth mentioning, as they provide alternative ways to think about policy features and their implications for evidence use. For example, Matland (1995) has developed an 'ambiguity-conflict' model which describes political issues in terms of their level of uncertainty and their level of contestation. This model was developed to consider the political resources required to improve policy implementation in different cases, but we can clearly see parallels in our discussions of complexity and contestation that could inform thinking on the use of evidence. Hisschemöller and Hoppe (2001) alternatively describe policy problems depending on whether there is consensus on the relevant norms and values at stake, and certainty about the relevant knowledge to apply to solve the problem. They use a four-way classification system, seeing problems as: structured; moderately structured in terms of the *ends*; moderately structured in terms of the *means*; and unstructured. Shaxson (2009) has built on Hisschemöller and Hoppe's framework by linking it more directly with complexity concepts from Snowden and Boone (2007) to reflect on how the way in which a problem is structured (badly, well, partially or unstructured) has implications for the relationship between science and policy – e.g. with science 'leading' policy in structured cases, providing only one of many voices in some unstructured cases, or helping to shape debates in 'badly' structured situations. These alternative frameworks can thus provide additional insights and ways of thinking about the relationship between science and policy. Yet here our choice ultimately reflects the desire to develop a system that allows for more direct engagement with the political origins of evidentiary bias.

Conclusion

This chapter has explored how the origins of many sources of bias lie in the inherently competitive nature of policy debates. However, the idea that policy arenas may *inherently* incentivise biased uses of evidence may be disconcerting to those who believe that faithful uses of scientific evidence can and should work to improve social outcomes. Of importance to this audience is to recognise that having a better understanding of the political origins of various forms of bias can also enable reflection on strategies to mitigate them. So, for example, Bacchi criticises the EBP movement for its failure to recognise how political problems are rhetorically constructed in ways that dictate which evidence is seen to be relevant, but in response, she has developed a set of questions that can be used by policy analysts to make problem constructions more visible, directly asking what the problem is represented to be, what is excluded from the representation, how the problem representation can be questioned, etc. (Bacchi 2012). Oreskes and Conway, on the other hand, who discuss the strategies corporate actors use to undermine science, have alternatively recommended the scientific community to pursue particular approaches, such as building consensus and increasing the clarity of messages, to counter the 'merchants of doubt' who promote uncertainty around issues such as climate change (Oreskes and Conway 2010).

And there are a range of other potential approaches that might mitigate one or more manifestations of bias identified in this chapter. For example, when programme officials are incentivised to 'cheat' to show better results, governments can establish rules or practices that separate those who measure success of programmes from those who stand to benefit from them (e.g. having schools not test their own pupils or not hold their own students' answer sheets). Alternatively, when there is widespread pressure for the 'uptake' of selective pieces of research evidence, governments can establish official knowledge-brokering bodies that can serve as entry points for researchers to present their findings, working to include evidence across a range of considerations in policy debates.

Some of these possible responses can be embodied in government bureaucratic structures. Others may be 'best practices' that can be embraced by researchers, technical advisors, the media or the public. Still others may reflect changes in rules and practice over how evidence is created or provided to inform decision making. The potential list of strategies is vast and Chapter 8 will return to these examples and others in its discussion on the need to build institutional structures, rules and norms that can help to address the origins and manifestations of bias. However, before this, we next turn to a second way in which politics can manifest in bias – not through the overt pursuit of political interests, but through more subtle unconscious cognitive processes.

References

Bacchi, Carol. 2009. *Analysing Policy: What's the Problem Represented to Be?* Frenchs Forest NSW: Pearson Australia.

——. 2012. 'Introducing the "what's the problem represented to be?" approach'. In *Engaging with Carol Bacchi: Strategic Interventions and Exchanges*, edited by Angelique Bletsas and Chris Beasley, pp. 21–24. Adelaide: University of Adelaide Press.

Baumgartner, Frank, Jeffrey Berry, Marie Hojnacki, Beth Leech and David Kimball. 2009. *Lobbying and Policy Change: Who Wins, Who Loses, and Why*. Chicago: University of Chicago Press.

Baumgartner, Frank and Beth Leech. 1998. *Basic Interests: The Importance of Groups in Politics and in Political Science*. Princeton: Princeton University Press.

BBC News. 2015. 'Indian government failing to publish UN health report'. http://www.bbc.co.uk/news/world-asia-india-33375754, accessed 23 June 2016.

Beckett, Lois. 2013. 'America's most outrageous teacher cheating scandals'. http://www.propublica.org/article/americas-most-outrageous-teacher-cheating-scandals, accessed 23 June 2016.

Bero, Lisa A. 2005. 'Tobacco industry manipulation of research'. *Public Health Reports* 120(2): 200–208.

Blinder, Alan. 2015. 'Atlanta educators convicted in school cheating scandal'. *New York Times*, 1 April. http://www.nytimes.com/2015/04/02/us/verdict-reached-in-atlanta-school-testing-trial.html, accessed 23 June 2016.

Brooke, John Hedley. 1991. *Science and Religion: Some Historical Perspectives*. Cambridge: Cambridge University Press.

Brown, Sophie. 2015. 'DWP block release of figures on number of people dying after benefits stopped'. *Huffington Post*, 12 June. http://www.huffingtonpost.co.uk/2015/06/11/statistics-refused-benefits-death_n_7561918.html, accessed 23 June 2016.

Cartwright, N. and J. Hardie. 2012. *Evidence-Based policy: A Practical Guide to Doing it Better*. Oxford: Oxford University Press.

Chen, Stephen. 2015. 'Most Chinese cities hiding vital pollution data from public'. *South China Morning Post*, 29 March. http://www.scmp.com/news/china/article/1202211/most-chinese-cities-hiding-vital-pollution-data-public, accessed 23 June 2016.

Chew, Sarah, Natalie Armstrong and Graham Martin. 2013. 'Institutionalising knowledge brokering as a sustainable knowledge translation solution in healthcare: How can it work in practice?' *Evidence & Policy: A Journal of Research, Debate and Practice* 9(3): 335–351. doi: 10.1332/174426413X662734.

Davies, Huw, Sandra Nutley and Peter Smith. 2000. *What Works? Evidence-Based Policy and Practice in Public Service*. Bristol: Polity Press.

DeLeon, Peter. 2006. 'The historical roots of the field'. In *The Oxford Handbook of Public Policy*, edited by Michael Moran, Martin Rein and Robert E. Goodin, pp. 39–57. Oxford: Oxford University Press.

Dobbins, Maureen, Paula Robeson, Donna Ciliska, Steve Hanna, Roy Cameron, Linda O'Mara, Kara DeCorby and Shawna Mercer. 2009. 'A description of a knowledge broker role implemented as part of a randomized controlled trial evaluating three knowledge translation strategies'. *Implementation Science* 4(1): 23. doi: 10.1186/1748-5908-4-23.

Easton, David. 1971 [1953]. *The Political System: An Inquiry into the State of Political Science*. New York: Alfred A. Knopf.

Fischer, Frank. 2003. *Reframing Public Policy*. Oxford: Oxford University Press.

Fischer, Frank and John Forrester. eds. 1993. *The Argumentative Turn in Policy Analysis and Practice*. Durham, NC: Duke University Press.

Fleegler, E. W., L. K. Lee, M. C. Monuteaux, D. Hemenway, and R. Mannix. 2013. 'Firearm legislation and firearm-related fatalities in the United States'. *JAMA Internal Medicine* 173(9): 732–740. doi: 10.1001/jamainternmed.2013.1286.

Freedman, Des. 2006. 'Dynamics of power in contemporary media policy-making'. *Media, Culture & Society* 28(6): 907–923.

Glouberman, Sholom and Brenda Zimmerman. 2002. *Complicated and Complex Systems: What Would Successful Reform of Medicare Look Like?* Toronto: Commission on the Future of Health Care in Canada.

Greenhalgh, Trisha and Jill Russell. 2009. 'Evidence-based policymaking: A critique'. *Perspectives in Biology and Medicine* 52(2): 304–318.

Hall, Shannon. 2015. 'Exxon knew about climate change almost 40 years ago'. *Scientific American.* http://www.scientificamerican.com/article/exxon-knew-about-climate-change-almost-40-years-ago, accessed 23 June 2016.

Hammersley, Martyn. 2013. *The Myth of Research-Based Policy and Practice*. London: Sage.

Heywood, Andrew. 2007. *Politics*. Basingstoke: Palgrave Macmillan.

Hickel, Jason. 2015. 'The hunger numbers: Are we counting right?' *The Guardian*, 17 July. http://www.theguardian.com/global-development-professionals-network/2015/jul/17/the-hunger-numbers-are-we-counting-right, accessed 23 June 2016.

——. 2016. 'The true extent of global poverty and hunger: Questioning the good news narrative of the Millennium Development Goals'. *Third World Quarterly* 37(5):749–767. doi: 10.1080/01436597.2015.1109439.

Hisschemöller, Matthijs and Rob Hoppe. 2001. 'Coping with intractable controversies: The case for problem structuring in policy design and analysis'. In *Knowledge, Power, and Participation in Environmental Policy Analysis*, edited by Matthijs Hisschemöller, Rob Hoppe, William Dunn and Jerry Ravetz, pp. 47–72. Piscataway: Transaction Publishers.

Hoppe, Robert. 2005. 'Rethinking the science-policy nexus: From knowledge utilization and science technology studies to types of boundary arrangements'. *Poiesis & Praxis* 3(3): 199–215.

Jacob, Brian A. and Steven D. Levitt. 2003. 'Rotten apples: An investigation of the prevalence and predictors of teacher cheating'. *Quarterly Journal of Economics* 118(3): 843–877. doi: 10.1162/00335530360698441.

Jasanoff, Sheila S. 1987. 'Contested boundaries in policy-relevant science'. *Social Studies of Science* 17(2): 195–230.

Jones, Jeffrey M. 2011. 'Record-low 26% in U.S. favor handgun ban'. http://www.gallup.com/poll/150341/Record-Low-Favor-Handgun-Ban.aspx?utm_source=genericbutton&utm_medium=organic&utm_campaign=sharing, accessed 23 June 2016.

Kurtz, Cynthia and David Snowden. 2003. 'The new dynamics of strategy: Sense-making in a complex and complicated world'. *IBM Systems Journal* 42(3): 462–483.

Langer, Laurenz, Janice Tripney and David Gough. 2016. *The Science of Using Science: Researching the Use of Research Evidence in Decision-Making*. London: EPPI-Centre, Social Science Research Unit, UCL Institution of Education, University College London.

Lasswell, Harold. 1971. *A Pre-view of Policy Sciences*. New York: American Elsevier Publishing.

——. 1990 [1936]. *Politics: Who Gets What, When and How*. Gloucester, MA: Peter Smith Publisher.

Lavis, John, Govin Permanand, Cristina Catallo and BRIDGE Study Team. 2013. *How Can Knowledge Brokering Be Advanced in a Country's Health System?* Copenhagen: WHO Regional Office for Europe.

Lerner, Daniel and Harold Dwight Lasswell. eds. 1951. *The Policy Sciences: Recent Developments in Scope and Method.* Stanford: Stanford University Press.

Levitt, Steven. 2005. 'The cheating curve: What are the costs of high-stakes testing?' http://www.chicagobooth.edu/capideas/may05/cheating.html, accessed 23 June 2016.

Liverani, Marco, Benjamin Hawkins and Justin Parkhurst. 2013. 'Political and institutional influences on the use of evidence in public health policy: A systematic review'. *PloS One* 8(10): e77404.

Mably, Paul. 2006. *Evidence-Based Advocacy: NGO Research Capacities and Policy Influence in the Field of International Trade.* Ottawa: International Development Research Center.

Matland, Richard. 1995. 'Synthesizing the implementation literature: The ambiguity-conflict model of policy implementation'. *Journal of Public Administration Research and Theory* 5(2): 145–174.

Mazzetti, Mark and Matt Apuzzoaug. 2015. 'Inquiry weighs whether ISIS analysis was distorted'. *New York Times*, 25 August. http://www.nytimes.com/2015/08/26/world/middleeast/pentagon-investigates-allegations-of-skewed-intelligence-reports-on-isis.html?_r=0, accessed 23 June 2016.

Myers, Matthew. 2013. 'The FCTC's evidence-based policies remain a key to ending the tobacco epidemic'. *Tobacco Control* 22(1): i45–i46. doi: 10.1136/tobaccocon trol-2012-050891.

Nutley, Sandra, Isabel Walter and Huw Davies. 2007. *Using Evidence: How Research Can Inform Public Services*. Bristol: Policy Press.

Oliver, Kathryn, Simon Innvar, Theo Lorenc, Jenny Woodman and James Thomas. 2014. 'A systematic review of barriers to and facilitators of the use of evidence by policy-makers'. *BMC Health Services Research* 14(1): 1–12. doi: 10.1186/1472-6963-14-2.

Oliver, Kathryn, Theo Lorenc and Simon Innvaer. 2014. 'New directions in evidence-based policy research: A critical analysis of the literature'. *Health Research Policy and Systems* 12(1): 34. doi: 10.1186/1478-4505-12-34.

Ongolo-Zogo, Pierre, John Lavis, Goran Tomson and Nelson Sewankambo. 2014. 'Initiatives supporting evidence informed health system policymaking in Cameroon and Uganda: A comparative historical case study'. *BMC Health Services Research* 14(1): 612. doi: 10.1186/s12913-014-0612-3.

Oreskes, Naomi. 2004. 'Science and public policy: What's proof got to do with it?' *Environmental Science & Policy* 7(5): 369–383.

Oreskes, Naomi and Erik Conway. 2010. 'Defeating the merchants of doubt'. *Nature* 465(7299): 686–687.

——. 2011. *Merchants of Doubt: How a Handful of Scientists Obscured the Truth on Issues from Tobacco Smoke to Global Warming.* London: Bloomsbury Publishing.

Parsons, Wayne. 2002. 'From muddling through to muddling up: Evidence-based policy making and the modernisation of British government'. *Public Policy and Administration* 17(3): 43–60. doi: 10.1177/095207670201700304.

Pielke, Roger A. 2002. 'Science policy: Policy, politics and perspective'. *Nature* 416(6879): 367–368.

Russell, Bertrand. 1997. *Religion and Science*. New York: Oxford University Press.

Rutter, Aclice, Benjamin Hawkins and Justin Parkhurst. 2013. *Knowledge Transfer and Exchange: A Look at the Literature in Relation to Research and Policy*. London: GRIP-Health Programme.

Sabatier, Paul A. 1988. 'An advocacy coalition framework of policy change and the role of policy-oriented learning therein'. *Policy Sciences* 21(2): 129–168. doi: 10.1007/bf00136406.

——. ed. 2007. *Theories of the Policy Process*, 2nd edn. Boulder: Westview Press.

Schön, Donald A. and Martin Rein. 1994. *Frame Reflection: Toward the Resolution of Intractable Policy Controversies*. New York: Basic Books.

Shaxson, Louise. 2009. 'Structuring policy problems for plastics, the environment and human health: Reflections from the UK'. *Philosophical Transactions of the Royal Society: Biological Sciences* 364(1526): 2141–2151.

Smith, Katherine. 2013. *Beyond Evidence-Based Policy in Public Health: The Interplay of Ideas*. Basingstoke: Palgrave Macmillan.

Snowden, David J. and Mary E. Boone. 2007. 'A leader's framework for decision making'. *Harvard Business Review* 85(11): 68–76.

Snyder, S. 2013. The simple, the complicated, and the complex: Educational reform through the lens of complexity theory. In *OECD Education Working Papers*. Paris: OECD Publishing.

Stone, Deborah. 2002. *Policy Paradox: The Art of Political Decision-Making*. London: W.W. Norton.

Stout, Lynn A. 2008. 'Why we should stop teaching Dodge v. Ford'. *Virginia Law & Business Review* 3: 163–176.

Susskind, Lawrence. 2006. 'Arguing, bargaining, and getting agreement'. In *Oxford Handbook of Public Poilicy*, edited by Michael Moran, Martin Rein and Robert Goodin, pp. 269–295. Oxford: Oxford University Press.

Thomas, Charlie. 2013. 'Cigarette giant JTI's plain packaging advert banned after government policy claim found to be false'. *Huffington Post*, 13 March. http://www.huffingtonpost.co.uk/2013/03/11/cigarette-giant-jtis-plain-packaging_n_2851860.html, accessed 23 June 2016.

Ulucanlar, Selda, Gary J. Fooks, Jenny L. Hatchard and Anna B. Gilmore. 2014. 'Representation and misrepresentation of scientific evidence in contemporary tobacco regulation: A review of tobacco industry submissions to the UK government consultation on standardised packaging'. *PLoS Medicine* 11(3): e1001629. doi: 10.1371/journal.pmed.1001629.

UNICEF. 2010. *Advocacy Toolkit: A Guide to Influencing Decisions that Improve Children's Lives*. New York: United Nations Children's Fund.

Van Kammen, Jessika, Don de Savigny and Nelson Sewankambo. 2006. 'Using knowledge brokering to promote evidence-based policy-making: The need for support structures'. *Bulletin of the World Health Organization* 84: 608–612.

Vogell, Heather. 2011. 'Investigation into APS cheating finds unethical behavior across every level'. http://www.ajc.com/news/news/local/investigation-into-aps-cheating-finds-unethical-be/nQJHG, accessed 23 June 2016.

Ward, Vicky, Allan House and Susan Hamer. 2009. 'Knowledge brokering: The missing link in the evidence to action chain?' *Evidence & Policy: A Journal of Research, Debate and Practice* 5(3): 267–279.

Weiss, Carol H. 1979. 'The many meanings of research utilization'. *Public Administration Review* 39(5): 426–431.

——. 1991. 'Policy research: data, ideas, or arguments'. In *Social Sciences and Modern States: National Experiences and Theoretical Crossroads*, edited by Peter Wagner, Carol Hirschon Weiss, Björn Wittrock and Hellmut Wollmann, pp. 307–332. Cambridge: Cambridge University Press.

Wesselink, Anna, Hal Colebatch and Warren Pearce. 2014. 'Evidence and policy: Discourses, meanings and practices'. *Policy Sciences* 47(4): 339–344. doi: 10.1007/s11077-014-9209-2.

WHO. 2012. *Evidence-Based Advocacy: Opportunities for Countdown to 2015 in Asia-Pacific*. Geneva: WHO.

5 The subtle politics of evidence

The cognitive-political origins of bias

> [T]he human understanding is like a false mirror, which, receiving rays irregularly, distorts and discolors the nature of things by mingling its own nature with it.
>
> Francis Bacon (1620)

While the preceding chapter discussed the origins of evidentiary bias that arise from the pursuit of political interests within a fundamentally competitive policy arena, this chapter explores a second, less immediately observable, origin of bias. Here we particularly draw on the field of cognitive psychology to explore the ways in which common, yet often unconscious, mental processes may also induce technical and issue bias. As will be shown, many of these instances can be directly linked to our existing values and beliefs, thus making them political in origin. Yet these biases may be less easily recognisable than those explored in the previous chapter and can thus be termed the *subtle* politics of evidence.

Human cognition: a missing explanatory link?

The field of cognitive psychology has developed rapidly over the past few decades in its investigation and description of how the human mind processes information. Within this field, there is often reference made to two different modes of cognition, referred to as 'System 1' and 'System 2' thinking, or what Daniel Kahneman (2011) has popularised as 'thinking fast' and 'thinking slow'. System 1 captures automatic and intuitive judgements about information we encounter, made unconsciously without voluntary control, while System 2 captures the controlled conscious mental activities demanding deliberate effort, for instance, in undertaking calculations or solving complex problems. Reliance on fast thinking can lead to particular errors, such as the selection of intuitive, but inaccurate, answers to problems. Yet, particularly when situations of uncertainty arise, the human mind has been shown to rely on a number of simplifying 'heuristics', even when more conscious or deliberate calculations are being made (De Martino et al. 2006; Kahneman and Tversky 1974; Sternberg 1996).

The utilisation of these (often unconscious) heuristics to aid judgement can themselves result in a set of associated biases (Gilovich and Griffin 2002).

The term 'bias' in this literature refers to a broad range of errors in information processing that diverge from classic ideas of 'rational' decision making. These include the inaccurate assessment of statistics or probability data, such as people's tendencies to over-estimate the risk of dying from rare diseases and under-estimate the risk of death from more common causes (Lichtenstein et al. 1978), but they further include tendencies towards other errors such as stereotyping, selective information review, drawing premature conclusions, and constructing erroneous causal explanations (Baron 2000; Gilovich, Griffin and Kahneman 2002; Kahneman 2011).

In recent years, we have begun to see a range of authors applying these insights to social issues as well, including to the popular understandings of science and public thinking about politics. Ben Goldacre, for instance, dedicates a chapter of his book *Bad Science* (2010) to the question of 'why clever people believe stupid things', in which he describes how cognitive processes help explain phenomena such as public belief in medical hoaxes, misunderstandings of health data or faith in disproven solutions (like homeopathy). George Lakoff (2008) and Drew Westen (2007), on the other hand, have both applied cognitive theories to understand political thinking in the US, reflecting on how political argumentation, and the public's processing of politically relevant information, is likely to be biased by our existing beliefs and affinities.

Of course, despite the modern growth and application of the cognitive sciences, the quote at the start of this chapter illustrates that there has been a much longer recognition that humans can be prone to errors. Writing in the early seventeenth century, Francis Bacon described a number of common human tendencies to perceive information inaccurately in his *Novum Organum Scientarium* [*New Instrument of Science*]. He defines a set of four 'Idols' that capture aspects of biased human perception:

- The *Idols of the Tribe* – reflecting tendencies to distort or exaggerate information.
- The *Idols of the Cave* – including errors based on prejudices arising from past experiences.
- The *Idols of the Marketplace* – capturing the ambiguity of meaning within words and language.
- The *Idols of the Theatre* – encompassing false learning embedded in philosophies or religions that are taken without question (Bacon 1908 [1620]; see also Hall undated).

Bacon's *Novum Organum* has been described as laying some of the key foundations to the scientific method in its discussions of logic and means to discovering truth, providing one of the early contributions to the 'Age of Enlightenment' that took hold in the seventeenth and eighteenth centuries (*New World Encyclopedia* 2015). Yet while the ideals of the scientific method are still widely espoused, Lakoff (2008) has noted that some other ideas from this era may be more problematic. In particular, he has taken issue with the 'Enlightenment view' of human reasoning based in the '18th century brain'. Specifically, he critiques the way in which human reasoning was believed to be fundamentally conscious, logical, unemotional and value-neutral – a perception that still endures today, explaining:

> If this were right, politics would be universally rational. If the people are made aware of the facts and figures, they should naturally reason to the right conclusion . . . [but] Enlightenment reason does not account for real political behaviour because the Enlightenment view of reason is false.
>
> (Lakoff 2008, p. 8)

However, the idea that evidence can, or should, be understood and utilised 'rationally' remains an implicit assumption behind many calls for evidence-based policymaking today. As such, there remains a large gap in our efforts to apply our knowledge of human cognition to the problems of evidence use for policy-making. This gap was similarly identified by the US National Research Council, which reviewed the use of scientific knowledge in public policy and concluded that while:

> There is an extensive literature in cognitive social psychology and behavioral decision theory on how people make judgments, decisions, and choices . . . These sciences have not . . . been applied to collective reasoning and group decision making *in public policy settings* at anything close to the level needed.
>
> (National Research Council 2012, p. 57, emphasis in original)

This chapter attempts to address this gap by exploring how cognitive heuristics and biases may explain a number of instances of technical and issue bias described previously. It further considers the political nature of these cognitive sources in terms of how they derive from value positions we hold and how they play out in competitive policy arenas. The chapter then works to build a 'cognitive-political model of evidentiary bias' that considers how the nature of different political issues may be likely to engender in one form of evidentiary bias or another, given the understandings of origins of bias outlined in both this and the preceding chapter.

Policy-relevant heuristics and biases

The policy process often involves making choices about which courses of action to follow in specific settings, with reference to multiple competing social values and concerns. Typically, this is also done in time-constrained circumstances and may be based on complex or partial information being available. Described in this way, a number of common simplifying heuristics can be identified that would be particularly relevant to explain how individuals understand and use scientific evidence within such environments, such as:

- The *availability heuristic*, which describes when decision making is aided by reliance on the memory of similar cases or the ease with which similar situations come to mind (Schwarz and Vaughn 2002),
- *Attribute substitution*, defined by Kahneman as 'when confronted with a difficult question people often answer an easier one instead, usually without being aware of the substitution' (2002, p. 53).
- The *representativeness heuristic*, which refers to cases where pieces of information are assumed to go together because we perceive similarity between a given situation and a prototypical (or stereotypical) one (Gilovich and Griffin 2002; Kahneman and Tversky 1974).
- The *affect heuristic*, which captures the process by which judgments are influenced by existing positive and negative ('affective') feelings (Finucane et al. 2000).

These heuristics are subsequently linked to a range of equally important biases including:

- *Illusory correlations*, described by Sternberg as where 'we tend to see particular events or particular attributes and categories as going together because we are predisposed to do so' (1996, p. 396).
- *Confirmation bias*, defined by Nickerson as 'the seeking or interpreting of evidence in ways that are partial to existing beliefs, expectations, or a hypothesis in hand' (1998, p. 175).
- *Cognitive dissonance aversion*, which refers to how individuals unconsciously avoid or reduce situations of 'dissonance' that arise when they are presented with information that leads to a conflict or contradiction between valued outcomes or ideas (Festinger 1962; Wicklund and Brehm 1976).

However, what is particularly important here for our purposes is to recognise that these heuristics and biases are often linked to our existing values and beliefs – things that are fundamentally at stake in political debates. As such, our political interests can work to predispose us towards biases in the use of policy-relevant evidence through cognitive processes which act to ensure that our values and beliefs remain unchallenged or undefeated, even in the face of potentially contradictory evidence. Yet, the unconscious nature of much of this cognitive bias makes it a much more *subtle* politics of evidence than the processes explored in the previous chapter arising from strategic choices made in the pursuit of political interests.

Motivated reasoning

One of the most well-known applications of the cognitive sciences has been in the field of behavioural economics, leading to investigations of how economic and behavioural choices can be influenced (or 'nudged') by a range of variables such as external cues, frames, anchors or other factors that neoclassical or rational choice economic theories might otherwise see as irrelevant to assessments of utility (cf. Mullainathan and Thaler 2000; Samson 2015; Thaler and Sunstein 2008).

Yet in this chapter, our interest lies more in policymaking arenas. Nevertheless, the field of political psychology is one of the few areas that have applied the heuristics and biases work directly to questions of how individuals understand political information. In doing so, authors have developed the term 'motivated reasoning' to capture some of the ways in which our pre-existing political affinities unconsciously lead to biased assessments of policy-relevant evidence (Kahan 2011; Kunda 1990; Redlawsk, Civettini and Emmerson 2010).

Many motivated reasoning insights have come from experimental studies. In one example, Redlawsk and colleagues (2010) undertook experiments to see how voters with a pre-existing preference for a candidate would respond to negative information about that candidate. They found that presenting prospective voters with a small amount of negative information led to their level of support going up rather than down – at least until a 'tipping point' was reached. The authors conclude that: 'Motivated reasoners strive to maintain existing evaluative affect, even in the face of countervailing information' (2010, p. 589).

In another example, Yeo et al. (2015) studied how a sample of Americans would respond to evidence about the relatively obscure field of nanotechnology – a subject for which they had little prior interest or knowledge – based on the source of information. The information was presented as coming either from Fox News (presumed to be conservative in its political orientation) or MSNBC (which had a perceived liberal orientation). The experiment found that participants on both sides of the liberal–conservative political spectrum demonstrated *defensive avoidance*, in which they avoided information when they believed the media source to be contrary to their political disposition, as well as *confirmation bias*, in which they searched for information from those sources felt to be congruent with their existing attitudes.

Other experiments have shown that existing political ideology can also lead to distrust of science or expertise more generally. Kahan (2014), for instance, found that that when individuals were asked to judge the level of expertise of a scientist (based on academic and professional qualifications), their judgement would be influenced by whether the expert presented statements that aligned or disagreed with their political beliefs. Similarly, Nisbet, Cooper and Garrett (2015) found that when subjects were presented with scientific information counter to their political views (e.g. presenting American conservatives with evidence of climate change or presenting liberals with evidence on the advantages of nuclear power), they later reported greater suspicion of the scientific community *as a whole*. Findings like this have led Kraft, Lodge and Taber to describe an unconscious 'hyperskepticism' towards scientific information by ideologues amongst both Republicans and Democrats in the US, arguing that 'these patterns can be understood as part of a general tendency among individuals to defend their prior attitudes and actively challenge attitudinally incongruent arguments' (2015, p. 121). Scientific denialism, as mentioned in the previous chapter, can therefore be understood not only as an overt strategy pursued to achieve particular interests, but as an unconscious intuitive response to situations where scientific evidence impinges on deeply held values.

Finally, motivated reasoning research also shows that it is not simply a lack of knowledge about a subject area or reliance on intuitive errors alone that drives the biased assessment of evidence. If this were the case, then provision of more knowledge or establishing contexts to ensure careful reflection would deal with all such errors. Instead, experiments have demonstrated situations where individuals with *increased* levels of knowledge on an issue, or individuals with *greater* scientific or numerical abilities, were *more likely* to interpret information in biased ways. Taber and Lodge (2006), for instance, showed that for two politically sensitive issues in the US (affirmative action and gun control), individuals with greater scientific knowledge demonstrated greater incidence of 'disconfirmation bias' – effectively using their abilities to search for information to counter-argue the facts or figures they disliked.

Kahan et al. (2013) also found that while more cognitively skilled individuals made fewer errors in interpreting numerical data about a politically neutral intervention (presented as the efficacy of a skin-rash cream), these individuals were *more likely* to come to erroneous (biased) conclusions when the same data were presented as the effectiveness of gun control policy. The authors explain this result as due to the process of 'identity protective cognition', in which individuals are motivated to use evidence in ways that are supported by their peer groups rather than by fidelity to evidence itself. Writing elsewhere, Kahan (2013) has given a further explanation of this phenomenon, stating that:

> shared ideological or cultural commitments are likely to be intertwined with membership in communities of one sort or another that furnish those individuals with important forms of support – emotional and psychic as well as material . . . If a proposition about some policy-relevant fact comes to be commonly associated with membership in such a group, the prospect that one might form a contrary position can threaten one's standing within it. Thus, as a form of 'identity self-defense', individuals are unconsciously motivated to resist empirical assertions . . . if those assertions run contrary to the dominant belief within their groups.
>
> (2013, p. 408)

Cognitive insights and the politics of evidence

The research on motivated reasoning summarised above has predominantly consisted of experiments with members of the public in the US, leading to Lodge and Taber (2013) developing what they have termed a 'John Q. Public' model of motivated reasoning. This model describes how the information processing of ordinary people follows unconscious steps heavily influenced by existing affective views and prior attitudes (see also Kraft, Lodge and Taber 2015). Yet, the work on heuristics, biases and motivated reasoning can provide insights into the origins of technical and issue bias not only in members of the public, but also in scientific experts, politicians and technical decision makers, as the following sections will explore.

Experts do it too: the case of the World Bank

In the early 1990s, James Ferguson (1994) critically analysed the policies of the World Bank's development programme in Lesotho, arguing that the approach of the programme was based on erroneous assessments of Lesotho's economy and infrastructure. Examples included incorrectly describing the economy as based on subsistence farming, stating that the country was reliant on exporting agricultural products rather than wage labour and selectively presenting statistics conducive to desired programme strategies. By comparing a range of original data sources to the World Bank's assessment of the country, Ferguson argues that 'these mistakes and errors are always of a particular kind, and they almost invariably tend in predictable directions. The statistics are wrong, but always wrong in the same way; the conceptions are fanciful, but it is always the same fantasy' (1994, p. 55). Ferguson concludes that Lesotho was being portrayed according to a stereotypical idea of a 'less developed' country, needing to be 'brought into the modern economy', as this concept fit with the World Bank's existing models of financial assistance and African development.

Ferguson's book describing this example has been a popular case study for students in the field of international development for over two decades, but what is particularly interesting is not just that the World Bank might have been biased in its assessment of evidence, but how that agency has recently reflected on its own biases. The annual World Development Report (WDR) is a flagship publication of the World Bank and, in 2015, the WDR was specifically dedicated to the topic of 'mind, society and behaviour', with a focus on human decision making and development policy. The report includes an overview of the field of cognitive psychology, reflecting on how social policy interventions can use behavioural insights to better achieve their goals. Examples include how regular reminders can improve adherence to medical treatments, how timing cash transfers to families at the time of school enrolment can increase the use of these to fund education or how a more intuitive provision of information can lead to more effective financial decisions in poor populations.

Yet a section of the WDR 2015 is also dedicated to discussing biases inherent within development professionals themselves, presenting results of a number of experiments undertaken with the World Bank's own staff to explore how they are affected by heuristics and biased thinking. So, for example, the organisation replicated Kahan et al.'s (2013) experiment on the interpretation of data depending on whether it was presented as showing the effectiveness of either skin-rash cream or gun control policy, but they replaced the gun control scenario with one of minimum wage policy. They confirmed that, just as with members of the American public, their professional staff were also less likely to interpret the data accurately when it was framed as measuring minimum wage policy effectiveness. This was particularly influenced by the pre-existing views that staff members had on the importance of income inequality as a social concern (World Bank 2015, p. 182). The report ends up identifying a range of biases and errors demonstrated in World Bank staff, including confirmation bias, sunk cost bias and inaccurate predictions of the beliefs of the poor people that they are meant to be serving with their work. The report even discusses some of its failures in the Lesotho programme described by Ferguson 20 years earlier, explaining that the mental models of the development professionals failed to take account of some of the key features of the local economy (2015, p. 187).

Shared values and particularly subtle politics of evidence

Much of the experimental research on motivated reasoning described earlier is based on research subjects who disagree over fundamental political values (e.g. liberals and conservatives in America). Yet the World Bank experience appears to illustrate that biases linked to affective positions can occur when political values are shared. These instances of bias are still political, as they derive from our values and belief systems, yet they can be *particularly subtle*, or go unnoticed, due to the common nature of the views out of which they originate. This can potentially explain the instances of erroneous conclusions about the sources of HIV prevention success in Africa described in Chapter 3, for example. That chapter gave examples of Uganda and Senegal's HIV successes attributed to illusory correlations with particular policy responses (i.e. the early, inclusive, policy response in Senegal or the multisectoral policy in Uganda), with Senegal's case further demonstrating representativeness errors when it was assumed Senegal would naturally have had a higher prevalence rate, as was occurring in some other regions in Africa.

However, it is quite possible that these errors have their origins in cognitive biases such as affective reasoning. At the time, global health officials working in the field of HIV/AIDS held particularly strong beliefs about the benefits of particular political responses, as there was concern over the stigmatisation of HIV/AIDS and national denial of HIV epidemics (cf. UNAIDS 2000, 2002). As such, it would be quite natural – indeed, *intuitive* – from these affective positions to assume that Senegal's low prevalence must have been due to its political response or that Uganda's prevalence declines must have been due to the widely promoted multisectoral approach, even if these correlations were illusory. Yet, the fact that these values were shared in the global community means that the intuitive tendency to this bias would have been particularly common, and particularly subtle, with resultant errors persisting over time (Parkhurst 2013).

Another example of this within the global HIV/AIDS community can be seen in the long-held assumption that poverty drives the spread of HIV in low-income settings (cf. Leroy, Ruel and Verhofstadt 2009; Muntaner 1999; Wodak and Cooney 2005). This is a commonly heard statement, yet it has been shown to be an oversimplification of the epidemiological realities in most cases. Chin (2007), for instance, has illustrated that higher-income African countries tend to have higher HIV prevalence, while Parkhurst (2010) has illustrated that it is wealthier individuals in several low-income African countries who show the highest HIV prevalence rates. These findings may appear counter-intuitive and, indeed, when they have been presented to public health Master's degree students (from this author's personal experiences), some have initially looked for reasons why the data must be wrong. However, such a response is natural for an intelligent, but affectively directed, mind, reflecting Taber and Lodge's (2006) findings of 'disconfirmation bias' amongst scientifically sophisticated individuals. When we have strong affective feelings on an issue (as public health Master's degree students will inevitably have when discussing HIV prevention and poverty), we instinctively use our skills to counter 'attitudinally incongruent' evidence (such as data showing HIV associated with wealth).

Deeper analysis helps to understand the more complex relationships between wealth, poverty and HIV infection in low-income countries. HIV, of course, does not spread directly through having money (or not having money). Rather, there are aspects of wealthy lifestyles that can lead to HIV risk – for example, by living in urban areas with a higher background HIV prevalence or by being more mobile and linking to wider sexual networks (cf. Deane, Parkhurst and Johnston 2010; Lurie et al. 2003). There are equally aspects of poverty that lead to HIV risk – for example, when women must rely on transactional sex in situations of food insecurity (cf. Weiser et al. 2007). These social drivers are also likely to change over time. Just as smoking and obesity-related illness first affected wealthy individuals in many countries before transitioning to the poor, HIV/AIDS may also follow a similar trend as lifestyles change. The realities are clearly complex and at times uncertain, but as the heuristics and biases work so often shows, individuals are particularly prone to biased judgements of information in situations of complexity or uncertainty.

Some might question if such biases are important when our values are shared, asking does it matter if we only focus on the poverty-related risks of HIV, considering we widely agree that both poverty reduction and HIV reduction are worthy goals? The answer to this, of course, lies in Chapters 1 and 2, and the reasons for all the calls for improved evidence to inform policy in the first place. Poor evidence use risks ineffective or even harmful outcomes. In this case, if we attempted to prevent HIV by focusing on reducing poverty or if we blindly assumed that poverty reduction reduces HIV risk, we are likely to be unsuccessful in our goals and to miss the fact that some individuals brought out of poverty will face changing lifestyles that present new risks of infection. This is not to say that we should leave people in poverty for the sake of HIV prevention – that would be a fairly inexcusable moral position. But a more technically valid understanding of the evidence, achieved by overcoming our cognitive biases, can allow us to instead consider other options, such as how to mitigate HIV risk as part of poverty reduction programmes (see Parkhurst (2012) for a greater discussion of social values and HIV prevention).

Politicians misleading themselves

If members of the public and scientific experts alike demonstrate evidence of subtle politics biasing their use of evidence, we should not be surprised to see it in politicians as well. As the early chapters of this book established, evidence matters in policymaking because it can assist decision makers to achieve social goals. Yet some of the most egregious and well-known misuses and manipulations of evidence can be seen to come from politicians who should, in theory, be working to serve their populations. While the previous chapter explored how politicians may face political incentives (e.g. for re-election) leading to biased uses of evidence, there can equally be bias introduced through cognitive mechanisms amongst those entrusted to make decisions on behalf of the public.

One illustrative example of this can be to return to the example of Chapter 1 of the evidence justifying the 2003 war in Iraq. That chapter highlighted President George W. Bush's widely criticised claims of Iraqi efforts to build weapons of mass destruction. Yet the US was not the only country supporting the invasion using this (disputed) evidence base. The UK was equally supportive, with Prime Minister Tony Blair at the time stating: 'What I believe the assessed intelligence has established beyond doubt is that Saddam [Hussein] has continued to produce chemical and biological weapons, that he continues in his efforts to develop nuclear weapons, and that he has been able to extend the range of his ballistic missile programme' (*The Guardian* 2002).

Soon after the invasion, however, a key British report evaluated the intelligence evidence behind these claims, highlighting a number of weaknesses and problems with the evidence (Lord Butler of Brockwell 2004).* The author of the report, Lord Butler, was interviewed years later and asked how such problematic evidence could have led to such certainty, to which he responded that those involved 'misled themselves' (Taylor 2013). A similar explanation was also used by the former UN Weapons Inspector Hans Blix when he explained that he did not feel the Bush administration deliberately misled the public, but rather 'they misled themselves' (Tufts University 2005).

But what does this mean for politicians to 'mislead themselves' when evaluating evidence? The subtle politics of evidence explored in this chapter provides some potential explanations. Notably, both assessments (by Butler and Blix) concluded that the individuals involved were not *deliberately* trying to mislead. If deliberate, it would be a clear case of overt bias – strategic manipulation of evidence to achieve pre-set political goals. Instead, these assessments appear to indicate that the administrations were subject to unconscious errors, potentially including confirmation bias, illustrated by taking inconclusive evidence as 'proof' for a decision that was consonant with existing affinities or past experiences, e.g. pre-existing beliefs that Saddam Hussein was the type of person who was likely to work to obtain such weapons. Indeed, Blix further stated that the Bush administration 'were not critically thinking. They wanted to come to these conclusions' (Tufts University 2005).

Unconsciously biased towards 'what works'?

Finally, the cognitive sciences can also provide insights into the widespread, but often critiqued, embrace of the language of 'what works', and the deference to randomised controlled trials and hierarchies of evidence by some in the EBP movement. As explained in Chapter 2, there are some important problems with

* At the time this book was going to press, another report on the UK's participation in the war led by Sir John Chilcot was published, which again identified errors in the assessment of evidence in the lead up to the war. See: http://www.iraqinquiry.org.uk/.

the idea that we can simply follow evidence of 'what works' to guide policymaking. First, this fails to recognise that evidence of effect may not reflect the political priority of an intervention. Similarly, the 'what works' language can serve to marginalise more complex social policy goals and strategies – such as those dealing with disease prevention, long-term reductions in crime, holistic improvements in education, social change to improve gender equality, and the like – in lieu of more simplistic approaches such as managing the outcomes of these issues. The what works language also confuses the *internal* and *external validity* of research evidence – internal validity representing whether an intervention produced the result where it was done and external validity addressing whether it would produce the same result elsewhere (or specifically in a particular target policy context).

Sanderson has been critical of the reductionism to what works in the EBP movement by explaining that this thinking 'reflects the attractions of instrumental rationality as a response to the growing challenge of social complexity' (2009, p. 700). In many ways, then, equating policymaking with questions of 'what works' serves to replace the challenging, but essential, political question of 'what should we do in our situation?' with the simpler (more attractive) question of 'what produces an effect?' This replacement, however, can be seen to reflect Kahneman's (2002) description of attribute substitution – unconsciously substituting a complicated question with a more easily answerable one. As our discussion of issue bias has explored so far, there are genuine political implications of this substitution, because it can change where policy attention lies or which policy choices are prioritised.

Features of policy problems and mechanisms of bias

Just as in the previous chapter, which explored the origins of bias arising from the competitive pursuit of political interests, by understanding the unconscious mechanisms that manifest in bias, we can again find ourselves better positioned to expect when these may arise in policy arenas. Cognition may not be 'rational' (in the neoclassical economic sense), but as Ariely (2008) has stated, humans, and their cognitive errors, are in many ways 'predictably irrational'. In Chapter 4 we introduced how three key features of policy problems – the complexity of the issue, the level of contestation and the polarisation of the policy debate – could result in bias through overt mechanisms. We again use these features to reflect on how they may also engender bias through more subtle cognitive routes.

Complexity (and issue complication)

As before, it can be useful to utilise complexity theory's distinction between problems being *complicated*, when they involve multiple difficult, but solvable, elements, and when they are *complex*, involving some aspects of uncertainty (or even unsolvability). This is because each of these two types of problem may invoke the use of different heuristics and their associated biases. In difficult (complicated) cases, the problems may be answerable with sufficient evidence, but reliance on 'fast' thinking can still result in intuitive calculation errors, as well as other errors such as attribute substitution, representative bias or illusory correlation. As explored above, this may explain the instances of errors in the earlier discussions of AIDS in Africa, as 'slower' thinking could have potentially avoided some unfounded conclusions. In contrast, when faced with problems typified by *uncertainty*, thinking 'slow' cannot eliminate all unknowns, and other heuristics that deal with situations of partial information may still exist (Kahneman and Tversky 1974). The cognitive bias towards a distrust in science, for example, appears to be particularly relevant in cases where unknowns exist in policy-relevant science. Finally, having multiple social concerns at stake in complicated policy issues can increase the chances of affective reasoning on any one relevant concern, as well as the likelihood of situations of cognitive dissonance arising when values do not perfectly align between the multiple outcomes at stake.

Contestation/importance of the issue

The level of contestation over policy outcomes can obviously incentivise bias in overt ways, but the importance of a policy decision to an individual can also influence unconscious biases through what has been termed 'attitude strength' (Pomerantz, Chaiken and Tordesillas 1995). Studies have shown, for instance, that greater attitude strength can increase the utilisation of affective heuristics in particular, resulting in associated biases such as a greater misperception of risks or selective information gathering (Alhakami and Slovic 1994; Brannon, Tagler and Eagly 2007). High attitude strength may again help explain some of the examples of unconscious bias seen in the work of experts in the global health and development community. Individuals working in these fields have often chosen to do so because of strongly held values about social justice and a genuine desire to improve people's lives. Yet the stronger our convictions, the more susceptible we may be to particular affective biases – even for expert professionals. Finally, attitude strength can also influence the intensity of cognitive dissonance felt when evidence does not align with values. This was seen by Taber and Lodge (2006), for instance, who found that stronger prior held beliefs on controversial subjects (i.e. gun control or affirmative action) would increase confirmation bias to avoid cognitive dissonance.

Polarisation

The motivated reasoning research on affective biases, along with that on 'identity protective cognition', which explores bias deriving from a desire to remain congruent with an existing affinity group, has further implications when policy issues are highly polarised. However, we can also distinguish between two features of polarisation: the polarisation of the policy issue on the one hand and the polarisation of the political environment on the other.

As described in the previous chapter, the polarisation *of a policy issue* can refer to how many possible policy options or compromise positions are available within a single policy decision. Polarisation *of the political environment*, on the other hand, would refer to how wide a spectrum of political viewpoints and positions is held within a society more broadly. Kahan, for instance, describes a 'ubiquity and ferocity of ideological conflicts over facts that turn on empirical evidence' (2013, p. 407) in the US, which he sees, in part, as due to the polarisation of American politics. Indeed, scholars have described a tendency for declining political agreement or middle ground between liberals and conservatives over time in the American political environment (Layman, Carsey and Horowitz 2006; Pew Reseach Center 2014), in contrast to some European countries, which may be governed by multi-party coalitions and, as such, are more typified by political bargaining and compromise (Laver and Schofield 1998).

A polarised *policy issue* (for example, that of abortion or gay marriage, in which there are only two possible choices) could engender technically biased uses of evidence because any evidence that is dissonant to a policy position would imply support for a radically extreme opposite choice – there is no middle ground. This could thus lead to greater negative affective feelings and increased disconfirmation bias. In a polarised *policy environment*, on the other hand, the influence of 'identity protective cognition' will be particularly strong, as individuals may find themselves in widely divided social and personal networks split along political lines. In such cases, any interpretation of evidence that is in disagreement with the affinity group risks more extreme social isolation or ostracism than would be the case in a political environment with a range of middle-ground political positions.

A highly polarised political environment would also be likely to show high levels of clustering of distinct sets of social concerns. This could engender issue bias from groups on either side of the debate as they present evidence internally consistent with existing views by only including issues belonging to their preferred cluster – so, for example, in US health care reform debates, liberals may present evidence of how proposed policies address equity or the needs of marginalised groups, as these are core values that they typically cluster around, while conservatives may present evidence relating to different concerns, such as government spending, individual choice, or the impact on employers.

A cognitive political model of evidentiary bias

Combining the insights in the previous chapter with those developed here allows a construction of what can be termed a *cognitive political model of evidentiary bias*. This model maps out the features of the policy problem discussed and how they can generate both technical and issue bias, recognising that the mechanisms that engender bias can be both overt and subtle. The development of such a model, summarised in Table 5.1 below, can be used both to predict when bias may arise as well as to help inform strategies to mitigate or potentially avoid instances of evidentiary bias.

Table 5.1 A cognitive-political model of evidentiary bias

Features of policy problems	*Example sources of technical bias*	*Example sources of issue bias*
Complexity: **a Complicated**	A complicated case with many elements can increase reliance on intuitive 'fast' thinking and heuristic-driven processes for shortcuts. These can result in biases such as inaccurate judgements of probability or drawing illusory correlations.	By being multifaceted, complicated policies can involve a larger number of social concerns. This can mean a higher chance that the evidence utilised excludes one or more relevant policy considerations.
b Uncertain	Uncertainty can drive heuristics that engender bias such as deferring to established preferences or past experiences which may not accurately address the current issue. It is easier to sow doubt as a strategy to advance a political position when there are more scientific unknowns.	In situations of uncertainty, there is a greater likelihood for attribute substitution to resolve the unconscious desire for certainty – e.g. pursuing what can be measured, not necessarily what is important.
Contestation	When issues are more important to stakeholders, there will be a diminished relative value of scientific accuracy compared to the political importance of the issue. Greater issue importance reflects increased 'attitude strength' – linked to stronger affective feelings driving bias and more intense instances of cognitive dissonance.	Greater importance of policy outcomes can shape which ones are selected to be included or excluded from programme evaluations. Greater importance of the issue can lead to stronger incentives to review evidence speaking to a limited (preferred) set of social concerns.
Polarisation: **a of the issue**	Polarised issues imply 'all or nothing' or 'winner takes all' outcomes. With no option for compromise, there can be greater incentives to manipulate evidence to 'win'.	Having more to lose may increase incentives to review evidence speaking to a limited (preferred) set of social concerns.
b of the political environment	A political environment with only two (or a few) divided political groupings can lead to stronger motivation for identity-protective cognition (greater importance to maintain group acceptance).	Polarised environments can reflect a clustering of values and concerns at extremes, which may lead to the selection of evidence talking to only those issues supported by one or another side.

Understanding the problem to identify solutions

There are some who feel that the hard-wired nature of cognitive bias and motivated reasoning destine us all to a life of political irrationality. Kraft and colleagues are particularly pessimistic, speculating that 'if science denial stems from motivated reasoning processes that are fundamental to our basic cognitive architecture, we may simply not have the capacity to separate the evaluation of facts and reasons in a policy dispute from our hopes for which way the evidence will point' (2015, pp. 130–131). They similarly refer to the work of Bargh (1999), who describes unconscious information processing as a 'cognitive monster' that is particularly hard to control. Others have argued that such biases present a critical challenge to the democratic ideal. Taber and Lodge, for instance, state that: 'From one perspective the average citizen would appear to be both cognitively and motivationally incapable of fulfilling the requirements of rational behaviour in a democracy' (2006, p. 767). Richey (2012) has asked if cognitive bias represents a 'death knell' for deliberative democracy due to how it can undermine the idealised form of rational debate seen as a prerequisite for democratic decision making.

Others, however, are more optimistic, with Sherman arguing that 'the controllability of such biases has been underestimated' (2008, p. 391). Indeed, there is evidence to believe that when sources of bias can be made visible and understood, they can be avoided or overcome at times. Lewandowsky et al. (2012), for example, describe how correcting misinformation has been found to entrench bias further in some experiments, but go on to discuss strategies that may work to offset this process in political debates. Bias offsetting has also been implemented in professional environments as well. In the medical profession, for example, cognitive biases leading to treatment errors have been addressed by formalising procedural checklists (Gawande and Lloyd 2010) or through the active consideration of alternative outcomes (Arkes 1981). Similarly, in the sport of professional basketball, evidence showing unconscious racial bias by referees was overcome by making them aware of the bias in the first place (Pope, Price and Wolfers 2015). Morewedge et al. (2015) alternatively found that training interventions could reduce multiple cognitive biases relevant to strategic intelligence analysis, while Kahneman and colleagues (2011) have devised a checklist to follow before making a 'big decision' to help make individuals consciously consider if they might be influenced by biasing tendencies such as the affect heuristic, self-interest or confirmation bias.

Indeed, this chapter's construction of a cognitive-political model of evidentiary bias aims to provide a more strategic position from which to identify where biases arise, so as to help consider the bias mitigation strategies that may be useful in evidence-informed policy arenas. So, for example, we can consider how to design deliberative spaces which serve to *depolarise* discussions, such as by encouraging direct consideration of challenging positions and creating 'safe spaces' for alternative views, or by ensuring appropriate heterogeneity in the makeup of deliberating stakeholders (Sunstein 1999). We can also consider how to *de-incentivise* the evaluation process in order to reduce the importance of the issue to individuals involved – e.g. by ensuring autonomy from political interference for evidence advisors or to reduce pressure to show results. It may be early to draw firm conclusions, but there is clearly a very large area for future work to develop and test strategies to mitigate the many forms of bias mapped out in the cognitive political framework in Table 5.1. However, understanding the political origins of bias in greater depth is an important first step in this task.

Conclusion

The previous chapter discussed the incentives for biased uses of evidence deriving from competition within policy arenas. This chapter complements this by exploring the subtle politics of evidence that drives bias through cognitive processes linked to our values and belief systems. It is of course not new to recognise that our values can affect our decisions in both conscious and unconscious ways. Awareness of human errors in judgement has been recorded for centuries, and political incentives or conflicts of interests driving strategic uses of evidence have long been recognised. Yet recent advances in the cognitive sciences provide even greater insights into the origins and mechanisms of cognitive bias, particularly in situations of complexity, uncertainty and conflicting motivations.

As much as evidence can help improve the quality and effectiveness of social policy, biased uses of evidence risk undermining these goals, leading to inefficient policy decisions as well as seeming intractability when debates are unable to get beyond contradictory claims about evidence (Schön and Rein 1994). Given all we now know about bias, it could be argued that many of these outcomes should no longer be accepted as inevitable. Indeed, we can argue that it is inexcusable for heads of state to 'allow themselves to be misled' or to 'not critically think' when considering policy decisions as profound as whether to go to war. Similarly, we know enough about the incentives driving the overt political manipulation of evidence that we should no longer be surprised when groups with strong incentives to do so are found to be 'cheating' or manipulating data. The importance of accurate evidence use to inform decisions about education, public safety, climate change, health care or military action is too important, and the state of knowledge is too well established, to continue to perpetuate the eighteenth-century 'Enlightenment thinking' assumption that we are naturally rational, or to accept a naïve idealism that evidence will always be respected and honoured. We are all subject to biases and are all subject to incentives, particularly when our values (or the things we value) are at stake. There is no need to continue drawing erroneous conclusions from data, pursuing ineffective policy options or perpetuating undesirable social outcomes based on ignorance of these well-established principles – neither from our scientific experts, nor from elected officials who shoulder the responsibility of public policymaking.

Avoiding evidentiary errors and mitigating biases in the ways in which evidence is used to inform public policy can therefore be seen as part of the broader goal of improving the use of evidence in policymaking and ultimately achieving the great potential for evidence use outlined in Chapter 2. However, fully realising this goal requires a consideration of a number of additional issues in order to take the next steps beyond the current approaches of the EBP movement. First, we need to consider what constitutes *good evidence for policy*, given the critique of oversimplified appeals to hierarchies of evidence. Second, we need to consider what constitutes a *good use of evidence* from a political perspective in terms of how multiple values or interests are considered in processes that are reliant on evidence. Finally, there is a need to consider how to institutionalise structures, rules, norms and practices that serve to improve evidence use in policymaking in these ways. Each of these questions is addressed in turn in the final chapters that make up Part III of this book. In combination, they serve to construct the idea of the *good governance of evidence* to help address the challenges and issues raised so far, describing a normative ideal in which unbiased, rigorous and relevant evidence is used to inform decisions that remain representative of, and accountable to, local populations.

References

Alhakami, Ali Siddiq, and Paul Slovic. 1994. 'A psychological study of the inverse relationship between perceived risk and perceived benefit'. *Risk Analysis* 14(6): 1085–1096.

Ariely, Dan. 2008. *Predictably Irrational*. New York: HarperCollins

Arkes, Hal R. 1981. 'Impediments to accurate clinical judgment and possible ways to minimize their impact'. *Journal of Consulting and Clinical Psychology* 49 (3): 323–330.

Bacon, Francis. 1908 [1620]. *Novum Organum*, edited by Joseph Devey. New York: P.F. Collier and Son.

Bargh, John A. 1999. 'The cognitive monster: The case against the controllability of automatic stereotype effects'. In *Dual-Process Theories in Social Psychology*, edited by Shelly Chaiken and Yaacov Trope, pp. 361–382. New York: Guilford Press.

Baron, Jonathan. 2000. *Thinking and Deciding*. Cambridge: Cambridge University Press.

Brannon, Laura, Michael Tagler and Alice Eagly. 2007. 'The moderating role of attitude strength in selective exposure to information'. *Journal of Experimental Social Psychology* 43(4): 611–617.

Chin, James. 2007. *The AIDS Pandemic: The Collision of Epidemiology with Political Correctness*. Oxford: Radcliffe Publishing.

De Martino, Benedetto, Dharshan Kumaran, Ben Seymour and Raymond Dolan. 2006. 'Frames, biases, and rational decision-making in the human brain'. *Science* 313 (5787): 684–687. doi: 10.1126/science.1128356.

Deane, Kevin, Justin Parkhurst and Deborah Johnston. 2010. 'Linking migration, mobility, and HIV'. *Tropical Medicine & International Health* 15(12): 1458–1463.

Ferguson, James. 1994. *The Anti-politics Machine: 'Development', Depoliticization and Bureaucratic Power in Lesotho*. Minneapolis: University of Minnesota Press.

Festinger, Leon. 1962. *A Theory of Cognitive Dissonance*, vol. 2. Stanford: Stanford University Press.

Finucane, Melissa L., Ali Alhakami, Paul Slovic and Stephen M. Johnson. 2000. 'The affect heuristic in judgments of risks and benefits'. *Journal of Behavioral Decision Making* 13(1): 1–17. doi: 10.1002/(sici)1099-0771(200001/03)13:1<1::aid-bdm333>3.0.co;2-s.

Gawande, Atul and John Bedford Lloyd. 2010. *The Checklist Manifesto: How to Get Things Right*. New York: Metropolitan Books

Gilovich, Thomas and Dale Griffin. 2002. 'Introduction – heruistics and biases: Then and now'. In *Heuristics and Biases: The Psychology of Intuitive Judgement*, edited by Thomas Gilovich, Dale Griffin and Daniel Kahneman, pp. 1–18. Cambridge: Cambridge University Press.

Gilovich, Thomas, Dale Griffin and Daniel Kahneman. eds. 2002. *Heuristics and Biases: The Psychology of Intuitive Judgement*. Cambridge: Cambridge University Press.

Goldacre, Ben. 2010. *Bad Science: Quacks, Hacks, and Big Pharma Flacks*. Toronto: McClelland & Stewart.

The Guardian. 2002. 'Full text of Tony Blair's foreword to the dossier on Iraq'. www.theguardian.com/world/2002/sep/24/iraq.speeches, accessed 29 June 2016.

Hall, Manly P. undated. 'The four idols of Francis Bacon & the new instrument of knowledge'. www.sirbacon.org/links/4idols.htm, accessed 29 June 2016.

Kahan, Dan M. 2011. 'What is motivated reasoning and how does it work?' *Science + Religion Today*. www.scienceandreligiontoday.com/2011/05/04/what-is-motivated-reasoning-and-how-does-it-work, accessed 29 June 2016.

——. 2013. 'Ideology, motivated reasoning, and cognitive reflection'. *Judgment & Decision Making* 8: 407–424.

——. 2014. 'Making climate-science communication *evidence*-based – all the way down'. In *Culture, Politics and Climate Change: How Information Shapes Our Common Future*, edited by Deserai A. Crow and Maxwell T. Boykoff, pp. 203–220. Abingdon: Routledge (Earthscan).

Kahan, Dan M., Ellen Peters, Erica Cantrell Dawson and Paul Slovic. 2013. 'Motivated numeracy and enlightened self-government'. *Yale Law School, Public Law Working Paper* (307).

Kahneman, Daniel. 2011. *Thinking, Fast and Slow*. London: Allen Lane.

Kahneman, Daniel and Shane Frederick. 2002. 'Representativeness revisited: Attribute substitution in intuitive judgment'. In *Heuristics and Biases: The Psychology of Intuitive Judgement*, edited by Thomas Gilovich, Dale Griffin and Daniel Kahneman, pp. 49–81. Cambridge: Cambridge University Press

Kahneman, Daniel, Dan Lovallo and Olivier Sibony. 2011. 'Before you make that big decision'. *Harvard Business Review* 89(6): 50–60.

Kahneman, Daniel and Amos Tversky. 1974. 'Judgement under uncertainty: Heuristics and biases'. *Science* 185(4157): 1124–1131.

Kraft, Patrick W., Milton Lodge and Charles S. Taber. 2015. 'Why people "don't trust the evidence": Motivated reasoning and scientific beliefs'. *Annals of the American Academy of Political and Social Science* 658(1): 121–133. doi: 10.1177/0002716214554758.

Kunda, Ziva. 1990. 'The case for motivated reasoning'. *Psychological Bulletin* 108(3): 480–498.

Lakoff, George. 2008. *The Political Mind: Why You Can't Understand 21st-Century Politics with an 18th-Century Brain*. New York: Viking.

Laver, Michael and Norman Schofield. 1998. *Multiparty Government: The Politics of Coalition in Europe*. Ann Arbor: University of Michigan Press.

Layman, Geoffrey C., Thomas M. Carsey and Juliana Menasce Horowitz. 2006. 'Party polarization in American politics: Characteristics, causes, and consequences'. *Annual Review of Political Science* 9(1): 83–110. doi: doi:10.1146/annurev.polisci.9.070204.105138.

Leroy, Jef, Marie Ruel and Ellen Verhofstadt. 2009. 'The impact of conditional cash transfer programmes on child nutrition: A review of evidence using a programme theory framework'. *Journal of Development Effectiveness* 1(2): 103–129. doi: 10.1080/19439340902924043.

Lewandowsky, Stephan, Ullrich K. H. Ecker, Colleen M. Seifert, Norbert Schwartz and John Cook. 2012. 'Misinformation and its correction continued influence and successful debiasing'. *Psychological Science in the Public Interest* 13(3): 106–131.

Lichtenstein, Sarah, Paul Slovic, Baruch Fischhoff, Mark Layman and Barbara Combs. 1978. 'Judged frequency of lethal events'. *Journal of Experimental Psychology: Human Learning and Memory* 4(6): 551–578.

Lodge, Milton and Charles S. Taber. 2013. *The Rationalizing Voter* Cambridge: Cambridge University Press.

Lord Butler of Brockwell. 2004. *Review of Intelligence on Weapons of Mass Destruction*. London: The Stationery Office.

Lurie, Mark N., Brian G. Williams, Khangelani Zuma, David Mkaya-Mwamburi, Geoff P. Garnett, Adriaan W. Sturm, Michael Sweat, D., Joel Gittelsohn and Salim S. Abdool Karim. 2003. 'The impact of migration on HIV-1 transmission in South Africa: A study of migrant and nonmigrant men and their partners'. *Sexually Transmitted Diseases* 30(2): 149–156.

Morewedge, Carey K., Haewon Yoon, Irene Scopelliti, Carl W. Symborski, James H. Korris and Karim S. Kassam. 2015. 'Debiasing Decisions: Improved Decision Making with a Single Training Intervention'. *Policy Insights from the Behavioral and Brain Sciences* 2(1): 129–140. doi: 10.1177/2372732215600886.

Mullainathan, Sendhil and Richard Thaler. 2000. *Behavioral Economics*. Cambridge, MA: National Bureau of Economic Research.

Muntaner, Carles. 1999. 'Invited commentary: Social mechanisms, race, and social epidemiology'. *American Journal of Epidemiology* 150(2): 121–126.

National Research Council. 2012. *Using Science as Evidence in Public Policy*, edited by Kenneth Prewitt, Thomas A. Schwandt and Miron L. Straf. Washington DC: National Academies Press.

New World Encyclopedia. 2015. 'Age of Enlightenment'. www.newworldencyclopedia.org/entry/Age_of_Enlightenment, accessed 29 June 2016.

Nickerson, Raymond S. 1998. 'Confirmation bias: A ubiquitous phenomenon in many guises'. *Review of General Psychology* 2(2): 175–220. doi: 10.1037/1089-2680.2.2.175.

Nisbet, Erik C., Kathryn E. Cooper and R. Kelly Garrett. 2015. 'The partisan brain: How dissonant science messages lead conservatives and liberals to (dis)trust science'. *Annals of the American Academy of Political and Social Science* 658(1): 36–66. doi: 10.1177/0002716214555474.

Parkhurst, Justin. 2010. 'Understanding the correlations between wealth, poverty and human immunodeficiency virus infection in African countries'. *Bulletin of the World Health Organization* 88: 519–526.

——. 2012. 'HIV prevention, structural change, and social values: The need for an explicit normative approach'. *Journal of the International AIDS Society* 15 (Supplement 1).

——. 2013. 'The subtle politics of AIDS: Values, bias, and persistent errors in HIV prevention'. In *Global HIV/AIDS Politics, Policy, and Activism*, edited by Raymond A. Smith, pp. 113–139. Santa Barbara, CA: Praeger.

Pew Reseach Center. 2014. *Political Polarization in the American Public*. Washington DC: Pew Research Center.

Pomerantz, Eva, Shelly Chaiken and Rosalind Tordesillas. 1995. 'Attitude strength and resistance processes'. *Journal of Personality and Social Psychology* 69(3): 408–419.

Pope, Devin, Joseph Price and Justin Wolfers. 2015. *Awareness Reduces Racial Bias*. Washington DC: Brookings Institution.

Redlawsk, David. 2002. 'Hot cognition or cool consideration? Testing the effects of motivated reasoning on political decision making'. *Journal of Politics* 64(4): 1021–1044.

Redlawsk, David, Andrew Civettini and Karen Emmerson. 2010. 'The affective tipping point: Do motivated reasoners ever "get it"?' *Political Psychology* 31(4): 563–593.

Richey, Mason. 2012. 'Motivated reasoning in political information processing: The death knell of deliberative democracy?' *Philosophy of the Social Sciences* 42(4): 511–542.

Samson, Alain. 2015. 'The behavioral economics guide 2015'. www.behavioraleconomics.com/BEGuide2015.pdf, accessed 29 June 2016.

Sanderson, Ian. 2009. 'Intelligent policy making for a complex world: pragmatism, evidence and learning'. *Political Studies* 57(4): 699–719.

Schön, Donald and Martin Rein. 1994. *Frame Reflection: Toward the Resolution of Intractable Policy Controversies*. New York: Basic Books.

Schwarz, Norbert and Leigh Ann Vaughn. 2002. 'The availability heuristic revisited: Ease of recall and content of recall as distinct sources of information'. In *Heuristics and Biases: The Psychology of Intuitive Judgement*, edited by Thomas Gilovich, Dale W. Griffin and Daniel Kahneman, pp. 103–119. Cambridge: Cambridge University Press.

Sherman, Jeffrey. 2008. 'Controlled influences on implicit measures: Confronting the myth of process-purity and taming the cognitive monster'. In *Attitudes: Insights from the New Implicit Measures*, edited by R. E. Petty, R. H. Fazio and P. Briñol, pp. 391–426. New York: Psychology Press.

Sternberg, Robert J. 1996. *Cognitive Psychology*. Fort Worth: Hardcourt Brace College Publishers.

Sunstein, Cass R. 1999. 'The law of group polarization'. *University of Chicago Law School, John M. Olin Law & Economics Working Paper* (91).

Taber, Charles and Milton Lodge. 2006. 'Motivated skepticism in the evaluation of political beliefs'. *American Journal of Political Science* 50(3): 755–769.

Taylor, Peter. 2013. 'Iraq: The spies who fooled the world'. www.bbc.com/news/uk-21786506, accessed 29 June 2016.

Thaler, Richard and Cass Sunstein. 2008. *Nudge: Improving Decisions about Health, Wealth, and Happiness*. New Haven: Yale University Press.

Tufts University. 2005. 'The road to democracy'. http://enews.tufts.edu/stories/381/2005/10/24/BlixBringsWMDInsightsToFletcher, accessed 29 June 2016.

UNAIDS. 2000. *Comparative Analysis: Research Studies from India and Uganda: HIV and AIDS-Related Discrimination, Stigmatization and Denial*. Geneva: UNAIDS.

——. 2002. *A Conceptual Framework and Basis for Action: HIV/AIDS Stigma and Discrimination*. Geneva: UNAIDS.

Weiser, Sheri, Karen Leiter, David Bangsberg, Lisa Butler, Fiona Percy-de Korte, Zakhe Hlanze, Nthabiseng Phaladze, Vincent Iacopino and Michele Heisler. 2007. 'Food insufficiency Is associated with high-risk sexual behavior among women in Botswana and Swaziland'. *PLoS Medicine* 4(10): 1589–1598.

Westen, Drew. 2007. *The Political Brain*. New York: Public Affairs.

Wicklund, Robert and Jack Williams Brehm. 1976. *Perspectives on Cognitive Dissonance*. Hillsdale, NJ: Lawrence Erlbaum Associates.

Wodak, Alex and Annie Cooney. 2005. 'Effectiveness of sterile needle and syringe programmes'. *International Journal on Drug Policy* 16: 31–44.

World Bank. 2015. *World Development Report 2015: Mind, Society, and Behavior*. Washington DC: World Bank.

Yeo, Sara, Michael Xenos, Dominique Brossard and Dietram Scheufele. 2015. 'Selecting our own science: How communication contexts and individual traits shape information seeking'. *Annals of the American Academy of Political and Social Science* 658(1): 172–191. doi: 10.1177/0002716214557782.

Part III

Towards the good governance of evidence

6 What is 'good evidence for policy'?

From hierarchies to appropriate evidence[1]

What is evidence for anyway?

It is perhaps worth revisiting some of the early discussions of the initial chapters of this book to reflect on the reasons as to why evidence is seen as important in policymaking in the first place. A number of claims have been made about the benefits of evidence, but perhaps the most common is to hold that more or better uses of evidence can improve decision making in terms of policy effectiveness and programme efficiency (cf. Coalition for Evidence-Based Policy 2015; UK Government 2013). From this conceptualisation, when used accurately and with fidelity to scientific best practices, evidence tells us 'what works' to achieve programme goals so as to obtain improved outcomes, to save valuable limited resources and to select effective solutions to social problems (see similar discussion in Dhaliwal and Tulloch 2012; Shaxson 2005). Yet the conceptualisation of policymaking as an exercise in technical problem solving and discussions of evidence which appear to remove political considerations have led to many criticisms of the EBP movement outlined in Chapter 2, including a failure to understand the decidedly contested nature of policymaking and the risk of imposing a de facto set of policy priorities through the promotion of particular types of evidence.

However, Sanderson (2009) has argued that the realities of the policy process need not resign us to accept political manipulation of evidence. Despite the robust critique of EBP, he argues that we should retain the pragmatic normative goal of using evidence to improve social policy outcomes, while also recognising the complexity of the policy process. But given the discussions so far, the pursuit of a decidedly normative vision requires explicit consideration of several concerns of both evidence champions and their critics alike. Incorporating ideas from both camps requires conceptualising *an improved use of evidence* as one that ensures fidelity to scientific good practices, that applies evidence to achieve social goals and that also ensures that evidence-informed policy decisions remain democratically representative of the public's values. Yet, this conceptualisation compels us to more directly ask a set of key questions about how we can judge what better

1 Several ideas presented here are adapted from a previous paper published in Parkhurst and Abeysinghe (2016).

evidence for policy would look like, as well as what a better use of evidence in policymaking would be. This chapter begins with the first of these questions, revisiting the nature of policy-relevant evidence and asking what constitutes *good evidence* for policymaking given these normative ideals. Chapter 7 then follows by addressing the question of 'what is the *good use of evidence*?' with a focus on the policymaking process itself.

Beyond gold standards

As Chapter 2 explained, one of the main conceptual holdovers from the field of evidence-based medicine has been the widespread, and often uncritical, embrace of so-called 'hierarchies of evidence' to judge the relevance of evidence to inform policy decisions – typically placing methodologies such as randomised controlled trials (RCTs) or meta-analyses at the top of such hierarchies and often referring to them as the 'gold standard' of evidence. However, that chapter noted that these hierarchies were principally designed to judge evidence of intervention effect, not necessarily to reflect policy importance or relevance per se. Previous chapters have also noted that confusing evidentiary rigour with policy importance further risks generating issue bias by serving to prioritise those policy concerns that happen to be conducive to experimental evaluation.

Even within the health sector, other social concerns such as affordability, acceptability, equity or human rights are often key concerns for policy consideration – yet these may not be conducive to study via experimental trials. As Glasziou, Vandenbroucke and Chalmers have succinctly noted, 'different types of question require different types of evidence' (2004, p. 39), which has led Petticrew and Roberts (2003) to propose a typology of evidence based on the type of question being addressed (acceptability of a health intervention, effectiveness, satisfaction, etc.) as an alternative to a single hierarchy for health planning (see also the discussion in Parkhurst and Abeysinghe 2016). Dobrow et al. have made similar observations, also reflecting on the need for health policy-relevant evidence to be applicable locally, explaining that: 'Interpretation of evidence must acknowledge the varying nature of evidence for different policy objectives, balancing existing emphasis on evidentiary quality with more sophisticated methods for assessing the generalizability of evidence' (2006, p. 1181).

However, if traditional hierarchies do not provide the right tools by which to measure all policy-relevant evidence (even in the health sector from which they developed), this begs the question of how else we can go about judging what constitutes good evidence for public policymaking more broadly. This needs to be considered further in light of the normative concerns outlined above: that science is used accurately, that evidence works to achieve social goals and that evidence is utilised through processes that do not undermine the democratic representation of social concerns.

A starting point to consider this question can be taken from an analysis of the use of science and technology to inform policymaking within the field of sustainable development. As part of a broad research programme, Cash et al. (2003) reflected on a set of case studies that each analysed the knowledge systems which were used to inform decisions on environmental sustainability across a range of countries and regions (ranging from southern Africa to the Arctic). The authors found that the effectiveness of science to inform policy rested on three key attributes – *credibility*, *salience* and *legitimacy* – explaining:

> Credibility involves the scientific adequacy of the technical evidence and arguments. Salience deals with the relevance of the assessment to the needs of decision-makers. Legitimacy reflects the perceptions that the production of information and technology has been respectful of stakeholders' divergent values and beliefs, unbiased in its conduct, and fair in its treatment of views and interest.
>
> (2003, p. 8086)

These findings provide a useful starting point to reflect on how to move beyond hierarchies of evidence to consider what constitutes both good evidence and the good use of evidence from a policy perspective. Good evidence for policy can be seen to capture the ideas of credibility and salience identified by Cash and colleagues, as these concepts broadly capture the EBP movement's normative principles of fidelity to science and usefulness in order to achieve social goals. The idea of legitimacy, on the other hand, would be fundamental to a conceptualisation of what is a *good use of evidence for policy*, as it reflects critical policy scholars' concerns that evidence-informed policy decisions remain democratically representative of multiple social interests. Cash et al.'s findings were empirically derived, but we can further complement and expand on these insights with deeper conceptual engagement as well. The next chapter will deal with the process of using evidence for policy, but here we will first turn to the concerns over the evidence itself.

The appropriateness of evidence for policy needs

There is obviously no point in using 'high quality' evidence that is not relevant to the policy considerations at hand. As such, the first aspect discussed here of what might constitute 'good evidence for policy' expands on Cash et al.'s concept of *salience* by drawing on three related disciplinary fields in order to develop a framework of what is termed the *appropriateness*[2] of evidence for policy needs. The first field utilised is that of policy studies, which understands politics as involving multiple competing concerns and allows explicit reflection on which bodies of evidence address the political concerns at stake. The second is that of

2 The term 'appropriateness' is one that has also been used in political science to describe the rule-based logic that is built into political institutions and shapes the political thinking of individuals on what is considered correct behaviour – the so-called 'logic of appropriateness' of March and Olsen (2006). This is a broader interpretation than applied here, but there is an overlap in terms of recognition that key concerns or principles will shape thinking on what should be done, thus driving subsequent behaviour. Indeed, the concept of a good governance of evidence defined in the final chapter similarly can also be seen as constructing a 'logic of appropriateness' for the use of evidence which can be built into evidence-to-policy institutional arrangements.

sociology (and the sociology of knowledge), which fundamentally questions the way we construct and define data, and allows reflection of whether evidence is created in ways that are useful for policy concerns. The final field is that of the philosophy of science, which explores the causality and generalisability of social interventions in depth and, as such, allows reflection of how well evidence can be applied within a particular policy context.

Policy studies: decisions involve multiple concerns

The field of policy studies has informed much of the thinking in this book so far and has already provided the first insight into the limitations of existing hierarchies to provide a measure of good evidence for policy. Specifically, this relates to the recognition that policymaking involves multiple concerns and that outcomes of interest are often contested (Heywood 2007; Lasswell 1990 [1936]; Stone 2002). This of course implies that there are likely to be multiple bodies of relevant evidence to consider, depending on which policy outcomes are deemed important.

Indeed, when Harold Lasswell (1970) described the idea of the 'policy sciences' in the 1970s as a problem-oriented way to study and address social issues, he noted that the first intellectual task involved in this exercise must be that of 'goal clarification'. Yet there are no shortages of examples where discussions of evidence within social policy fields fail on this first task – by not making explicit the goals desired or the ultimate objectives of the programme of work. For many authors, the increasing reliance on RCTs or evidence hierarchies to guide policymaking risks obscuring the fundamental issue of goal clarification even further, and an example of this can be seen in the case of international development policymaking, presented in Box 6.1 below.

Box 6.1 What is good evidence for development policy?

The field of international development provides a useful example to illustrate the importance of being clear on policy goals and on how the embrace of experimental evidence may risk obscuring these goals as well. The development community, like many other social policy fields, has seen an evidence revolution of sorts in the past decade. Growing from a recognition that a large amount of aid money may have been squandered on ineffective programmes in the past (Court, Hovland and Young 2005), we see increasing calls for development policy to be informed by research evidence, and for international aid to show evidence of effect. This has led to a range of international research bodies and global agencies now embracing the language of 'evidence-based' development policy, similarly reflected in the launch of the *Journal of Development Effectiveness* in 2009 with the aim 'to support evidence-based policy making to enhance development effectiveness' (Taylor and Francis Online 2015).

The discourse of evidence-based development policy has also been accompanied by a proliferation of efforts to undertake more rigorous evaluations of interventions done in the name of development, including the growing embrace of RCTs to test the effects of development interventions (Deaton 2009). Groups such as J-PAL (the Abdul Latif Jameel Poverty Action Lab) at the Massachusetts Institute of Technology and Innovations for Poverty Action have particularly established themselves as leaders in the field of development evaluation through their use of experimental methods to evaluate a wide range of interventions, including cash transfers to families, access to credit to farmers, grants or performance-based pay for school teachers, provision of mass deworming treatments, etc. (Innovations for Poverty Action undated, J-PAL undated).

There is, however, a critical difference between evaluating whether interventions produce a beneficial effect and answering the question of what is good evidence for *development* policy (and, as Chapter 5 noted, it risks falling into the trap of attribute substitution if these two questions are conflated). This is because there is a much larger debate in the development community over what, in fact, are the key outcomes of interest for development policy – or, more fundamentally, around the question of what international development *should* look like. Goal clarification in this field, is therefore particularly important.

For many development scholars, the answer relates to economics. A number of authors evaluating the impact of foreign aid, for instance, have equated the goal of development with that of *economic growth* (cf. Cassen 1986). Indeed, Collier and Dollar justify this approach by stating that 'poverty reduction is the central goal of aid programmes' (2001, p. 3). Others, however, have argued that economic growth should not be the sole aim of development. Amartya Sen's work provides an alternative conceptualisation of the goal of development as a process of expanding *freedoms* by enhancing human capabilities – working to establish situations where people have the choice of which personal and social goals to achieve (Sen 1990, 1999). Others have alternatively asked whether foreign aid improves *democracy* (Knack 2004) and more recent critics of development efforts have also raised concerns over *inequality* as a result of aid (Deaton 2013) or over aid perpetuating corruption by undermining the *responsibility of the state* for its own citizens (Moyo 2009).

Whatever one's position on what is important for development – growth, poverty reduction, equality, state responsibility, democracy or freedoms – these considerations must be made explicit if there is any chance for development policy to be well informed by evidence. Asking 'what works for development' requires some form of goal clarification. Experimental evaluations may be methodologically rigorous, but they often select a narrow set of outcome indicators to measure – telling us whether funding for schools improves enrolment or whether the provision of bednets reduces the number of cases of malaria, for example. Yet there is a broader question of whether 'development' is achieved by having foreign governments pay families to send their children to school or by having philanthropists hand out nets. RCT methods are not designed to evaluate those broader questions and their usefulness needs to be considered with respect to the broad goals at stake, not just in terms of the immediate impacts they are well purposed to evaluate.

In order to be able to judge whether evidence is 'good', then, the first question we must ask is if it is relevant to the goals or purposes of the policy itself. Graphically we can use a simple diagram to illustrate the fact that, of the entire field of evidence available, there will be a sub-set of evidence that can be judged to be relevant in this way, illustrated simply in Figure 6.1 below. It is worth noting that some evidence outside the smaller circle in Figure 6.1 will be of high quality or come from methods commonly held at the top of hierarchies of evidence. But this does not necessarily mean that it is evidence of great usefulness to the policy decision at hand.

Good practice in evidence-informed policymaking must therefore start by incorporating a principle of goal clarification – making relevant policy concerns explicit. Without a clear indication of these, it is impossible to say whether evidence is good, or not, from a policy perspective, and it opens the door to issue bias as evidence of effect related to any potential outcome of interest can be championed on the basis of quality alone.

Sociological perspectives: evidence is constructed (in more or less useful ways)

A second disciplinary perspective that can help to reflect on what evidence might be considered appropriate for policymaking is that of sociology. Sociologists of knowledge (or of science) have particularly noted how social norms, ideologies

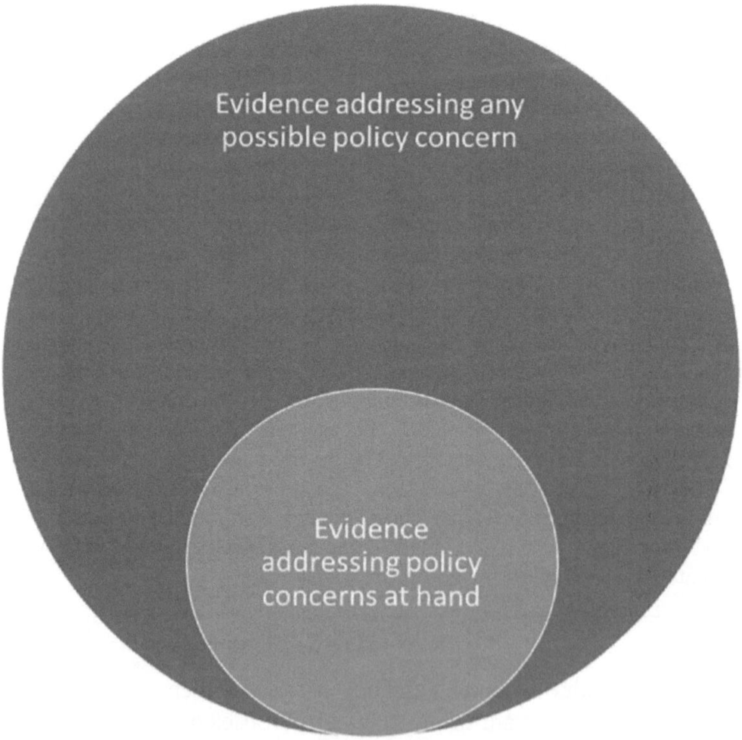

Figure 6.1 Evidence may or may not address the policy concerns at hand.

and power relations can be constructed into the creation of knowledge itself (cf. Bloor 1991; Longhurst 1989; Merton 1973) – describing data as a 'social product' (Krieger 1992, p. 413). As such, these perspectives recognise that what counts as evidence, including, for example, how variables are defined, will be a reflection of the culture or environment in which it is produced. The linked field of science and technology studies (STS) has further explored the dynamic boundaries between science and policy, illustrating that the ideas of what constitutes expertise, or what is seen as policy-relevant science, can actually be continually constructed and redefined throughout the policy process (cf. Gieryn 1999; Jasanoff 1987).

Many natural scientists and champions of EBP can find such concepts initially frustrating, as they appear to undermine the certainty of evidence or to challenge the foundations on which they base their reliance on evidence to justify action. Yet while epistemological differences no doubt present challenges across disciplines, from a normative perspective, based on the desire to use evidence to improve social welfare, these insights can actually provide a useful additional element to reflect on good evidence for policymaking. Fundamentally, they point to the fact that if evidence can be constructed in many possible ways (each of which may be judged technically valid), this provides a choice of how to construct and classify data based on the goals at hand.

So, for example, applied to health care, sociological perspectives have enabled a better understanding of how health outcomes arise from factors other than just biology. Krieger (1992) presents the example of Louis René Villermé, an epidemiologist working in Paris in the early 1800s, who recategorised data on mortality to explore the importance of neighbourhoods on health outcomes. While it is perhaps obvious today that neighbourhood residence can shape health, at the time, this fundamentally challenged ideas of how to study health determinants and helped open the door to a range of new public health policy options. More modern studies have similarly shown that patterns of health (or ill health) can be shaped through social relations related to gender (Courtenay 2000; Doyal 2000), ethnicity (Krieger et al. 2003) or class (Marmot and Wilkinson 2009; Wilkinson 2002). This perspective has led Krieger (1992) to note that the ways in which data are collected and reported will shape how problems are perceived, with important implications for the level of support or opposition that different programmes (i.e. policy responses) receive:

> Label infant mortality a problem of 'minorities' and present data only on racial/ethnic differences in rates, and the White poor disappear from view; label it as a 'poverty' issue and proffer data stratified only by income, and the impact of racism on people of colour at each income level is hidden from sight; define the 'race' or socioeconomic position of the infant solely in terms of the mother's characteristics, and the contributions of the father's traits and household class position to patterns of infant mortality likewise will be obscured.
>
> (1992, p. 412)

In these ways, the classification of population groups can affect both the support for policy action and the policy *options* available to the decision maker.

The field of HIV/AIDS prevention provides another example of this. It has been known for decades that a primary route of HIV transmission is through sexual contact. As such, it is clearly important to gather evidence about sexual practices in susceptible populations to help guide prevention efforts, and many low and middle-income countries take part in regular population health surveys that provide such information.[3] Yet for years, the sexual behaviour data collected in these surveys were limited to questions such as age at sexual initiation, number of past partners and use of a condom during the last sex act. However, over time, social epidemiologists and epidemiological modellers have questioned the usefulness of such evidence alone. So, for instance, it is recognised that HIV spreads more quickly through linked sexual networks and multiple concurrent sexual partners (Epstein and Morris 2011; Halperin and Epstein 2004). This recognition has led to some asking if we need changes to survey questions to attempt to capture concurrency data (Fishel, Ortiz and Barrère 2012) so as to inform more appropriate policy solutions to address this dynamic (Kalichman and Grebler 2010).

Sociologically informed approaches have further explained how sexual activity is not an individual characteristic, but rather a social phenomenon, with practices shaped at a group level (Hilber et al. 2012; Kippax, Holt and Friedman 2011; Kippax et al. 2013). Such an understanding allows alternative approaches to HIV prevention that address things like the social and structural drivers of risk practices (Seeley et al. 2012; AIDS2031 Social Drivers Working Group 2010). However, these new approaches need alternative evidence than what was provided in early surveys, requiring information about things like gender norms, economic drivers of sexual patterns or the social meanings associated with protected sex (Blankenship, Bray and Merson 2000; Parker, Easton and Klein 2000; Parkhurst 2014; Sumartojo 2000). In these ways, a critical reflection on the constructed nature of the evidence available may, in fact, open up greater policy options to achieve desired goals.

In Figure 6.2 (see following page), a similar figure to Figure 6.1 helps to illustrate how only a select range of evidence constructions will provide the most appropriate information for the policy goals at hand. As before, there will be constructions of evidence that rank highly in hierarchies of evidence that sit outside the small circle in this figure, but the lens of appropriateness would require first considering how useful the evidence is for particular goals.

Philosophy of science: generalisability and evidence in context

The philosophy of science provides a final perspective to help develop a conceptualisation of appropriate evidence. Some authors in this discipline have also identified that technical language on 'hierarchies of evidence' can obscure the political nature of policymaking (cf. Goldenberg 2006), but there is a particularly strong strand of work in this field that addresses the concepts of causality and

3 See http://www.dhsprogram.com for examples.

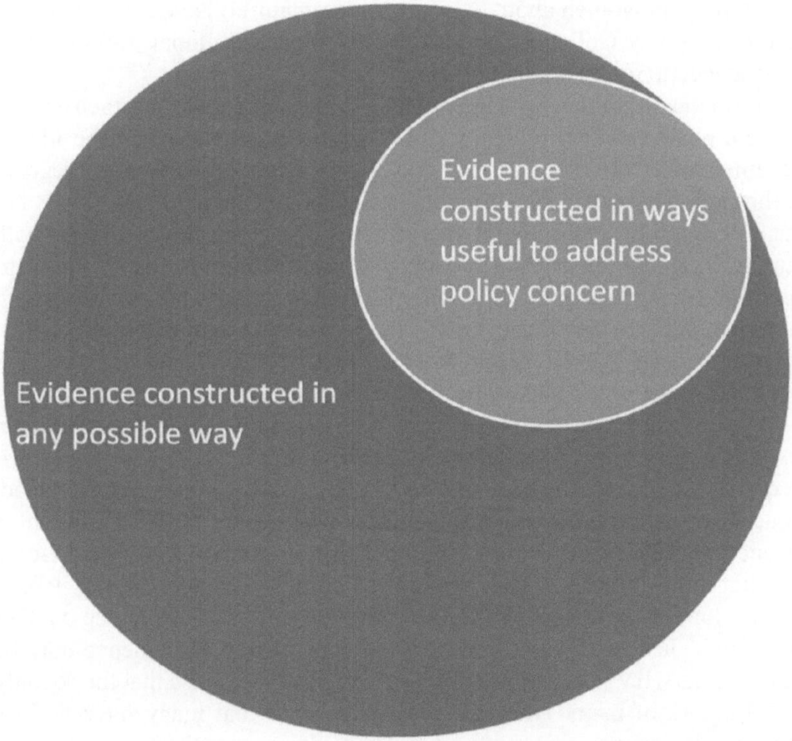

Figure 6.2 Evidence may be constructed in ways more or less useful for policy goals.

generalisability in evidence production as well. This captures the points noted in Chapter 2 in particular about the need to distinguish between the internal and external validity of evaluation studies – i.e. showing that an intervention that worked in one place does not necessarily mean that the intervention works *always* and *everywhere.* As Cartwright explains: 'For policy and practice we do not need to know "it works somewhere". We need evidence for "it-will-work-for-us"' (2011, p. 1401).

It was further explained in Chapter 2 that the generalisability assumed with most clinical trials arises from pre-existing knowledge about shared features of human biochemistry or anatomy, which provide the mechanisms through which clinical interventions produce a result. Yet the nature of the social world can be quite different, with interventions often working through alternative mechanisms in differing contexts (Cartwright 2011; Cartwright and Hardie 2012; Worrall 2010). This can be a particular challenge for the application of the method of meta-analysis to social concerns. Meta-analyses typically combine findings from multiple experiments to use a larger sample size than any one trial in order to have greater certainty of effect. It is a key tool promoted by the EBP movement, with a graphic presenting the results of a meta-analysis (on the use of corticosteroids in women about to give birth prematurely) even serving as the logo of the Cochrane Collaboration, the highly regarded global initiative that reviews evidence to guide clinical practice.

Yet systematically reviewing experimental trials and combining their results into a single point estimate typically relies on the assumption that the identical mechanism of effect exists across trials. Corticosteroids work in a pregnant woman through the same mechanisms in Tampa as in Timbuktu. Yet this is not necessarily the case for many social interventions. Chapter 2 illustrated this with the example of Robert Martinson's work that reviewed all published English-language reports on prisoner rehabilitation from a 20-year period and found 'no clear pattern to indicate the efficacy of any particular method of treatment' (1974, p. 49). Over two decades later, Pawson and Tilley (1997) noted that this was the most cited paper in the history of evaluation research and was widely interpreted as a conclusion that 'nothing works' for prison reform. Yet they explain that this study created 'an impossibly stringent criterion for "success"' (1997, p. 9), requiring studies to show impact across all included populations. Instead, they argue that it is more important to consider what works for whom in which circumstances, noting that the more useful conclusion to draw from Martinson's review is that 'most things have been found sometimes to work' (1997, p. 10).

We can return to the case of HIV prevention described above to see another example of this. Just as it was noted how the construction of evidence may be important to guide HIV prevention efforts, we can also recognise that the socially determined nature of many HIV risk practices means that many interventions might only work *sometimes*, requiring direct consideration of the mechanisms by which interventions have their effect in different contexts. A useful illustration of this comes in the form of recent experimental trials evaluating the provision of cash transfers to prevent HIV in African settings. Johnston has argued that cash transfers are a current fashion in Africa, 'liked by almost everyone, seemingly effective and potentially cheap' (2015, p. 409), yet she explains how evaluation of these programmes has shown particularly mixed results for HIV prevention. In some interventions, cash transfers resulted in lower HIV incidence (fewer new infections) compared to control groups, in others, it resulted in lower incidence for some but not all intervention sub-groups and in yet others, there was no significant difference for any groups (Johnston 2015). However, no doubt one of the main reasons for this is the simple fact that money will be used in different ways by people in different settings, which will only occasionally affect their HIV risk behaviours.

So, for instance, if women are reliant on selling sex to make ends meet, a cash transfer could conceivably reduce this high-risk practice. Yet in situations where having access to cash alternatively leads to broader social and sexual networking, this might inadvertently increase risk (Parkhurst 2010). Indeed, if a cash transfer was given to a population group known to routinely pay money for sex (such as travelling businessmen in some contexts), this could have the opposite effect to that intended on HIV risk behaviour.

A meta-analysis of cash transfers for HIV prevention might seem a good idea, but there would be little usefulness of any point estimate of impact found by combining the included studies. Systematically reviewing the literature may also be useful, but the lessons to learn from such a review would not come from assuming that the mechanism of effect is the same in all people. It is an over-simplified and erroneous question to ask 'do cash transfers work?'. Instead, reviews would need to look within studies to explore how the intervention was delivered and how it brought about an effect. Methods such as 'process evaluation' have grown in terms of their use to help investigate some of these elements (in particular, looking at which participants received particular components of interventions; Saunders, Evans and Joshi 2005) and alternatives such as 'realist evaluation' methods have developed to study mechanisms of intervention effect in different social contexts (Kazi 2003; Pawson and Tilley 1997). Evidence required for these sorts of questions do not necessarily make up the core features of experimental trials, but rather they supplement impact evaluations with additional methods such as in-depth qualitative or ethnographic analyses,

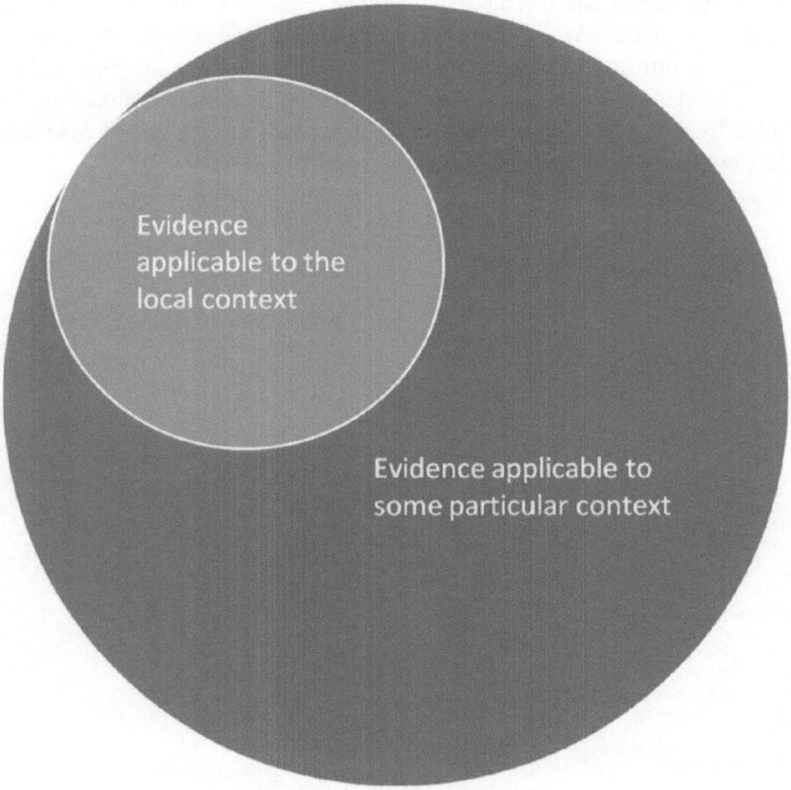

Figure 6.3 Evidence may be more or less applicable in the local policy context.

local surveys or quantitative sub-group analyses to generate evidence about mechanisms of effect. Such forms of evidence often rank low in existing hierarchies, but they may be particularly appropriate to the central policy question of: 'Will it work here?'

Returning to our simple graphics, Figure 6.3 is constructed to illustrate how bodies of evidence may be more or less relevant to the context addressed by the policy decision (see Figure 6.3 above). The figure particularly illustrates that there can be much evidence ranking highly on hierarchies in terms of quality that may not be applicable locally and, as such, may not be appropriate for the given policy needs.

From hierarchies to appropriateness

In combination, the three disciplinary perspectives drawn upon provide clear reasons why hierarchies of evidence, or single methods such as RCTs, should not be used as the sole measure of what constitutes 'good evidence for policy'. However, each perspective provides additional insights about which evidence best serves policy needs. A lens of appropriateness thus overlaps with Cash et al.'s (2003) definition of *salience*, requiring policy-relevant evidence to address the relevant policy concerns at stake, but our discussion above expands on this by identifying how appropriate evidence would further consist of evidence constructed in ways that are useful to inform those concerns and that is applicable to the local policy context. Appropriate evidence, then, can be illustrated by combining the smaller inner circles from the three figures above, representing the sub-set of evidence that captures when these elements overlap.

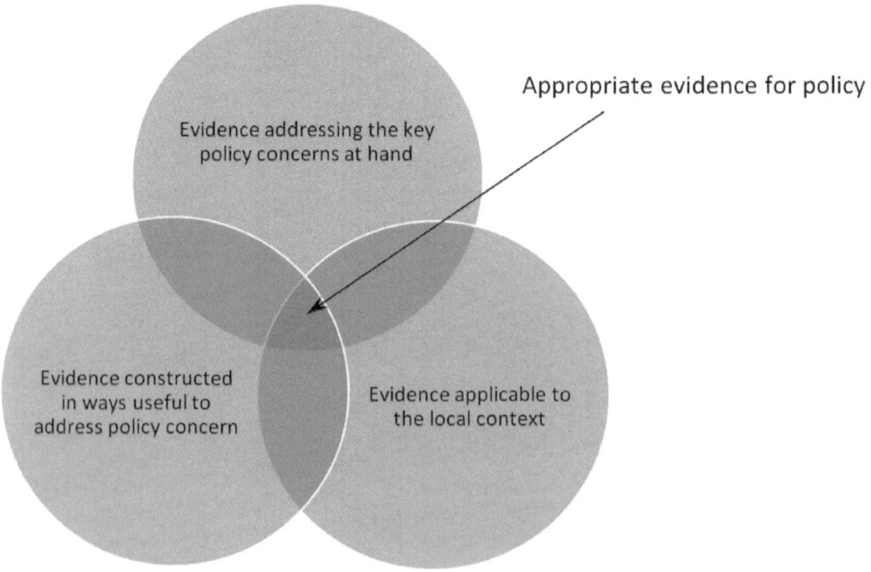

Figure 6.4 Appropriate evidence for policy context.

Doesn't quality matter?

The reader at this point might justifiably ask: but what about evidence *quality*? Indeed, this is the principal concern that hierarchies of evidence have been promoted to address. However, the discussion of appropriateness is not intended to diminish the importance of evidentiary quality, merely to supplement it. Simply put, quality does still matter, but the way to judge quality should be decided only after there is an identification of which evidence is most useful to the policy concern. The fact that certain forms of evidence will be more or less relevant to a policy issue does not mean that data variables are purely 'relative', with no way to judge between them. Rather, *methodological pluralism* is needed, an approach that is 'based on the principle of choosing the most suitable methods for the nature of the problem being researched' (Payne 2006, p. 174) and for which differing quality criteria will be relevant depending on the methodologies employed (Barker and Pistrang 2005; Dobrow et al. 2006).

So, for example, a relevant policy consideration for a decision maker could be the public acceptability of a course of action. Evidence to inform this would not rely on experimentation, but might instead involve survey methods. However, there are ways to undertake surveys in more (or less) rigorous ways. Surveys can be appropriate in terms of their sample size or underpowered. They can be biased in their selection of respondents or representative of the population. Similarly, another relevant policy concern might be the predicted costs over time. Appropriate evidence for this consideration may require economic modelling estimates, which in turn will have their own ways to evaluate quality and rigour.

Quality judgements can and should be used, but only after the sub-set of appropriate evidence is identified. The concern for quality of course overlaps with Cash et al.'s (2003) concept of *credibility,* defined as reflecting the 'scientific adequacy' of the technical evidence. And while in political debates there may be disagreement over which policy outcomes are most important, there can be agreement on the need for fidelity to scientific good practice for any given piece of evidence utilised. As Douglas has explained: 'While science is neither apolitical nor value-free, it can (and should) be pursued with integrity. Detecting science with integrity and defining the legitimate roles values play in such science opens the space for genuine deliberation and a way forward out of an ideological stalemate' (2015, p. 296).

Bringing the concern with quality and integrity back into our conceptualisation, then, *appropriate* evidence for policy can be seen to consist of evidence that addresses the political considerations at stake, that is constructed in ways that are useful to those considerations and that is applicable to the local policy context, while *good evidence for policy* can subsequently be defined as *appropriate evidence of high quality.* As noted, however, quality must be judged by the methodological principles relevant to the evidence base, as well as adherence to the broad principles of good scientific practices. So quality still matters, even if hierarchies of evidence do not provide the definitive measure of it in all cases.

Being systematic

One particular concern in evidence quality that is worthy of additional discussion is the importance of being systematic in gathering evidence to inform policy, particularly given the attention placed on systematic reviews as a tool to guide policy action. Being systematic and rigorous, as opposed to selective and piecemeal, is obviously an important part of scientific good practice for any investigation. Yet systematic reviews are a tool, just as RCTs are. They do not necessarily reflect good evidence for policy if they are not applied to the most relevant policy concerns or if their use obscures other important issues. Systematic reviews are also similar in some ways to meta-analyses in that they combine information from multiple sources, and they have been championed as better than single RCTs alone in terms of guiding choices between interventions (Chalmers, Hedges and Cooper 2002). But in their methods of combining information, they can at times risk stripping out political context and local concerns. This has led to Hammersley particularly critiquing the underlying assumptions behind systematic reviews, arguing that they may fail to provide useful knowledge in many cases (2013, Chapter 8).

Hammersley has been one of the most outspoken critics of the EBP movement, but as noted in the introductory chapters, this book is particularly interested in finding pragmatic ways forward from these debates. Doing so requires a realistic assessment of both the uses and limitations of different methodological techniques. Systematic reviews are one tool of evidence review that has developed to help answer particular questions. They do not address all policy-relevant issues and they may raise challenges of generalisability for many social policy problems, particularly if they focus solely on size of effect rather than on mechanisms of effect. But in their favour, they embed in their rules and norms some key principles of good scientific practice which should not be ignored. These include concerns over *transparency, replicability* and *comprehensiveness*, for instance, by listing explicitly how studies were found and how inclusion or exclusion criteria were used to review evidence (Gough, Oliver and Thomas 2012). Chalmers states quite clearly that systematic reviews need to be 'rigorous, transparent, and up to date' (2003, p. 33). These principles are important, even if systematic reviews, in their traditional form, do not address all the policy concerns at stake. The principle of *being systematic* – that is, being thorough, transparent, up to date and consistent in approach – is important to almost all forms of evidence generation and review. Indeed, these principles are embraced by newer methodologies being developed, such as 'realist review', which attempts to review literature on social interventions with explicit consideration of how mechanisms of effect work differently in different contexts (cf. McCormack et al. 2013; Pawson et al. 2005).

What about gaps in (policy-useful) evidence?

Perhaps a final caveat worth raising in this discussion of good evidence for policy is to recognise that good evidence for policy, as defined here, does not equate to evidence of absolute certainty. Of course, decision makers desire certainty (and as Chapter 5 points out, uncertainty can unconsciously drive particular biases), but in most real-world settings, many pieces of information of relevance to a decision may be unknown. Indeed, one of the biggest temptations of RCTs may be their allure of providing certainty from their ability to draw conclusions of causal effect. Yet only those interventions with simple and direct causal pathways will bring such certainty, and this still says nothing of the policy importance of that effect.

Some have argued that social policy is more often concerned with questions of a complex causal nature than of a simple direct nature (cf. Rittel and Webber 1973). Long-term and population-wide changes in education, health, crime, economic productivity and other fundamental social policy issues will all have multiple interacting determinants that are shaped by, or even created by, broader contextual factors like the physical environment in which one lives, social cohesion and norms, or the economic opportunities available. These realities can therefore result in gaps in knowledge on a regular basis. These realities have been highlighted by Davies and Nutley, who have explained:

> one observation is clear: the current state of research-based knowledge is insufficient to inform many areas of policy and practice. There remain large gaps and ambiguities in the knowledge base and the research literature is dominated by small, *ad hoc* studies, often diverse in approach, and of dubious methodological quality. In consequence, there is little accumulation from this research of a robust knowledge base on which policy makers and practitioners can draw.
>
> (2002, p. 6, emphasis in original)

As such, the authors argue that efforts for new knowledge creation must address a number of key issues, including identifying which research designs are appropriate for specific questions, balancing existing evidence versus new research, balancing rigour with timeliness, and a need to prioritise the gaps in knowledge relevant to policy decisions.

However, what this also means is that policy makers must often take action without perfect or complete information. In doing so, they may wish to choose policy options that are less certain, but that are judged more important, than lower-priority courses of action with greater predictability. In the field of health care, one example of this can be seen in the growing calls for policy action to address the social determinants of health (Commission on the Social Determinants of Health 2008; Marmot and Friel 2008). As Bonnefoy et al. (2007) explain, the relationship between social determinants and ultimate health outcomes 'is not precisely understood in causal pathway terms'. But, instead, they argue that: 'Although the precise causal pathways are not yet fully understood, enough is known in many areas, and the evidence is good enough, for us to take effective action' (2007, p. 11).

A judgement of when evidence is 'good enough' will be down to the individual decision maker, considering the importance of the issue and other trade-offs involved. But this provides another example of where a lens of appropriateness can help to guide policy action. The appropriateness framework is specifically shaped around policy needs and, as such, it allows more direct reflection on whether the existing evidence base (including any gaps) is useful *enough* when the goals and needs of the policy decision are explicitly considered.

Conclusions: a 'good evidence for policy' framework

While previous chapters raised concerns with technical and issue bias in the use of evidence and explored the political origins of these biases, this chapter provides the first contribution to the final section of the book by considering what constitutes good evidence for policy in the first place. In the field of environmental science, Cash et al.'s (2002) model of *credibility*, *salience* and *legitimacy* provides a starting point to reflect on this question. *Credibility* in many ways captures the well-established concerns over evidentiary quality, rigour and validity. But *salience* was seen as particularly critical in this chapter's discussion of what constitutes good evidence in terms of its policy relevance. It was illustrated that hierarchies of evidence cannot necessarily address this concern. Instead, this chapter drew on three disciplinary perspectives to further develop the concept of the appropriateness of evidence. The issue of quality was then re-introduced, specifically reflecting on the multiple methodological traditions that will generate policy-relevant evidence. In combination, these ideas can work to establish an understanding of what constitutes good evidence for policy, as illustrated in Figure 6.5 below.

Critically engaging with the question of what constitutes good evidence for policy does not abandon the previous section's interest in technical and issue bias. Indeed, in the framework presented on the following page, there is scope to acknowledge and accept the concerns of both sides of the EBP debate – with the need for evidence to address multiple social concerns while also adhering to principles of scientific best practice as well. It is clear from this perspective that RCTs and hierarchies of evidence provide appropriate evidence in some cases, but not in others. When the political concern is about impact of an intervention, then trials will indeed prove useful. But for many social policy decisions, reality is more complicated, and a lens of appropriateness may provide a way to recognise and act on this reality.

Policy is always adapting and changing, and policy considerations equally are continually in flux due to changing social interests and values. As such, there will be a continual need to clarify which evidence is more appropriate or most relevant to the policy issues at stake. However, a better understanding of what might be considered good evidence for policy is only one of the components needed to clarify how to improve the use of evidence in policymaking. Equally important is to think about what constitutes the good use of evidence from a policy perspective, to which we turn in the next chapter.

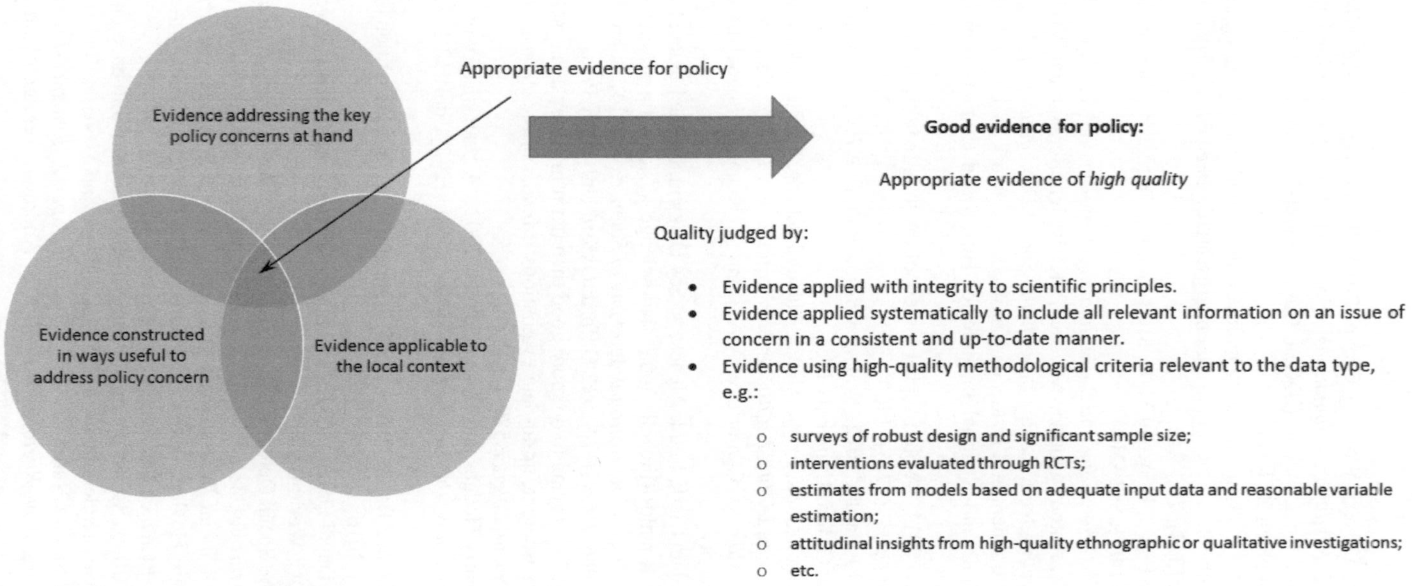

Figure 6.5 A conceptualisation of good evidence for policy.

References

AIDS2031 Social Drivers Working Group. 2010. *Revolutionizing the AIDS Response: Building AIDS Resilient Communities*. Worcester, MA: International Development, Community and Environment (IDCE), Clark University and International Center for Research on Women (ICRW).

Barker, C. and N. Pistrang. 2005. 'Quality criteria under methodological pluralism: Implications for conducting and evaluating research'. *American Journal of Community Psychology* 35(3–4): 201–212.

Blankenship, K. M., S. J. Bray and M. H. Merson. 2000. 'Structural interventions in public health'. *AIDS* 14(1): S11–21.

Bloor, David. 1991. *Knowledge and Social Imagery*. Chicago: University of Chicago Press.

Bonnefoy, Josiane, Antony Morgan, Michael P. Kelly, Jennifer Butt and Vivian Bergman. 2007. *Constructing the Evidence Base on the Social Determinants of Health: A Guide*. London: Measurement and Evidence Knowledge Network (MEKN), Universidad del Desarrollo, Chile and National Institute for Health and Clinical Excellence, United Kingdom.

Cartwright, Nancy. 2011. 'A philosopher's view of the long road from RCTs to effectiveness'. *The Lancet* 377(9775): 1400–1401.

Cartwright, N and J Hardie. 2012. *Evidence-Based Policy: A Practical Guide to Doing it Better*. Oxford: Oxford University Press.

Cash, David, William Clark, Frank Alcock, Nancy Dickson, Noelle Eckley and Jill Jäger. 2002. *Salience, Credibility, Legitimacy and Boundaries: Linking Research, Assessment and Decision Making*. Cambridge, MA: John F. Kennedy School of Government, Harvard University.

Cash, David, William Clark, Frank Alcock, Nancy Dickson, Noelle Eckley, David Guston, Jill Jäger and Ronald Mitchell. 2003. 'Knowledge systems for sustainable development'. *Proceedings of the National Academy of Sciences* 100(14): 8086–8091.

Cassen, Robert. 1986. *Does Aid Work?* Oxford: Oxford University Press.

Chalmers, Iain. 2003. 'Trying to do more good than harm in policy and practice: The role of rigorous, transparent, up-to-date evaluations'. *Annals of the American Academy of Political and Social Science* 589(1): 22–40.

Chalmers, Iain, Larry Hedges and Harris Cooper. 2002. 'A brief history of research synthesis'. *Evaluation & the Health Professions* 25(1): 12–37. doi: 10.1177/016327870 2025001003.

Coalition for Evidence-Based Policy. 2015. 'Our mission'. http://coalition4evidence.org, accessed 1 July 2016.

Collier, Paul and David Dollar. 2001. *Development Effectiveness: What Have We Learnt?* Washington DC: World Bank.

Commission on the Social Determinants of Health. 2008. *Closing the Gap in a Generation: Health Equity through Action on the Social Determinants of Health. Final Report of the Commission on Social Determinants of Health*. Geneva: World Health Organization.

Court, Julius, Ingie Hovland and John Young. 2005. *Bridging Research and Policy in Development: Evidence and the Change Process*. Rugby: ITDG.

Courtenay, Will. 2000. 'Constructions of masculinity and their influence on men's well-being: a theory of gender and health'. *Social Science and Medicine* 50(10): 1385–1402.

Davies, Huw and Sandra Nutley. 2002. *Discussion Paper 2: Evidence-Based Policy and Practice: Moving from Rhetoric to Reality*. St Andrews: Research Unit for Research Utilisation, University of St Andrews.

Deaton, Angus. 2013. *The Great Escape: Health, Wealth, and the Origins of Inequality.* Princeton: Princeton University Press.

Dhaliwal, Iqbal and Caitlin Tulloch. 2012. 'From research to policy: Using evidence from impact evaluations to inform development policy'. *Journal of Development Effectiveness* 4(4): 515–536.

Dobrow, Mark, Vivek Goel, Louise Lemieux-Charles and Nick Black. 2006. 'The impact of context on evidence utilization: A framework for expert groups developing health policy recommendations'. *Social Science & Medicine* 63(7): 1811–1824.

Douglas, Heather. 2015. 'Politics and science: Untangling values, ideologies, and reasons'. *Annals of the American Academy of Political and Social Science* 658(1): 296–306. doi: 10.1177/0002716214557237.

Doyal, Lesley. 2000. 'Gender equity in health: Debates and dilemmas'. *Social Science and Medicine* 51(6): 931–940.

Epstein, Helen and Martina Morris. 2011. 'Concurrent partnerships and HIV: An inconvenient truth'. *Journal of the International AIDS Society* 14(1): 13. doi: 10.1186/1758-2652-14-13.

Fishel, Joy, Ladys Ortiz and Bernard Barrère. 2012. *Measuring Concurrent Sexual Partnerships: Experience of the MEASURE DHS Project to Date.* Calverton, MD: ICF International.

Gieryn, Thomas. 1999. *Cultural Boundaries of Science: Credibility on the Line*. Chicago: University of Chicago Press.

Glasziou, Paul, Jan Vandenbroucke and Iain Chalmers. 2004. 'Assessing the quality of research'. *British Medical Journal* 328(7430): 39–41.

Goldenberg, Maya J. 2006. 'On evidence and evidence-based medicine: Lessons from the philosophy of science'. *Social Science & Medicine* 62(11): 2621–2632.

Gough, David, Sandy Oliver and James Thomas. 2012. *An Introduction to Systematic Reviews*. London: Sage.

Halperin, Daniel T and Helen Epstein. 2004. 'Concurrent sexual partnerships help to explain Africa's high HIV prevalence: Implications for prevention'. *The Lancet* 364(9428): 4–6.

Hammersley, Martyn. 2013. *The Myth of Research-Based Policy and Practice*. London: Sage.

Heywood, Andrew. 2007. *Politics*. Basingstoke: Palgrave Macmillan.

Innovations for Poverty Action. undated. 'Search studies'. http://www.poverty-action.org/search-studies, accessed 1 July 2016.

J-PAL. undated. 'Policy lessons'. https://www.povertyactionlab.org/policy-lessons, accessed 1 July 2016.

Jasanoff, Sheila S. 1987. 'Contested boundaries in policy-relevant science'. *Social Studies of Science* 17(2): 195–230.

Johnston, Deborah. 2015. 'Paying the price of HIV in Africa: Cash transfers and the depoliticisation of HIV risk'. *Review of African Political Economy* 42(145): 394–413.

Kalichman, Seth and Tamar Grebler. 2010. 'Reducing numbers of sex partners: Do we really need special interventions for sexual concurrency?' *AIDS and Behavior* 14(5): 987–990. doi: 10.1007/s10461-010-9737-5.

Kazi, Mansoor. 2003. 'Realist evaluation for practice'. *British Journal of Social Work* 33(6): 803–818. doi: 10.1093/bjsw/33.6.803.

Kippax, Susan, Martin Holt and Samuel Friedman. 2011. 'Bridging the social and the biomedical: Wngaging the social and political sciences in HIV research'. *Journal of the International AIDS Society* 14(2): S1.

Kippax, Susan, Niamh Stephenson, Richard Parker and Peter Aggleton. 2013. 'Between individual agency and structure in HIV prevention: Understanding the middle ground of social practice'. *American Journal of Public Health* 103(8): 1367–1375. doi: 10.2105/AJPH.2013.301301.

Knack, Stephen. 2004. 'Does foreign aid promote democracy?' *International Studies Quarterly* 48(1): 251–266. doi: 10.1111/j.0020-8833.2004.00299.x.

Krieger, Nancy. 1992. 'The making of public health data: Paradigms, politics, and policy'. *Journal of Public Health Policy* 13: 412–427.

Krieger, Nancy, Jarvis Chen, Pamela Waterman, David Rehkopf and S.V. Subramanian. 2003. 'Race/ethnicity, gender, and monitoring socioeconomic gradients in health: A comparison of area-based socioeconomic measures – the public health disparities geocoding project'. *American Journal of Public Health* 93(10): 1655–1671.

Lasswell, Harold. 1970. 'The emerging conception of the policy sciences'. *Policy Sciences* 1(1) :3–14.

——. 1990 [1936]. *Politics: Who Gets What, When and How*. Gloucester, MA: Peter Smith.

Longhurst, Brian. 1989. *Karl Mannheim and the Contemporary Sociology of Knowledge*. Basingstoke: Macmillan.

March, James and Johan Olsen. 2006. 'The logic of appropriateness'. In *The Oxford Handbook of Public Policy*, edited by Michael Moran, Martin Rein and Robert Goodin, pp. 689–708. Oxford: Oxford University Press.

Marmot, Michael and Sharon Friel. 2008. 'Global health equity: Evidence for action on the social determinants of health'. *Journal of Epidemiology and Community Gealth* 62(12): 1095–1097.

Marmot, Michael and Richard Wilkinson. 2009. *Social Determinants of Health*. Oxford: Oxford University Press.

Martin Hilber, Adriane, Elise Kenter, Shelagh Redmond, Sonja Merten, Brigitte Bagnol, Nicola Low and Ruth Garside. 2012. 'Vaginal practices as women's agency in Sub-Saharan Africa: A synthesis of meaning and motivation through meta-ethnography'. *Social Science & Medicine* 74(9): 1311–1323. doi: 10.1016/j.socscimed.2011.11.032.

Martinson, Robert. 1974. 'What works? Questions and answers about prison reform'. *The Public Interest* 35(2): 22–54.

McCormack, Brendan, Joanne Rycroft-Malone, Kara DeCorby, Alison Hutchinson, Tracey Bucknall, Bridie Kent, Alyce Schultz, Erna Snelgrove-Clarke, Cheyl Stetler, Marita Titler, Lars Wallin and Valerie Wilson. 2013. 'A realist review of interventions and strategies to promote evidence-informed healthcare: A focus on change agency'. *Implementation Science* 8(1): 107. doi: 10.1186/1748-5908-8-107.

Merton, Robert K. 1973. *The Sociology of Science: Theoretical and Empirical Investigations*. Chicago: University of Chicago Press.

Moyo, Dambisa. 2009. *Dead Aid*. London: Penguin.

Parker, R. G., D. Easton and C. H. Klein. 2000. 'Structural barriers and facilitators in HIV prevention: A review of international research'. *AIDS* 14(1): S22–32.

Parkhurst, Justin. 2010. 'Understanding the correlations between wealth, poverty and human immunodeficiency virus infection in African countries'. *Bulletin of the World Health Organization* 88: 519–526.

——. 2014. 'Structural approaches for prevention of sexually transmitted HIV in general populations: Definitions and an operational approach'. *Journal of the International AIDS Society* 17(1). doi: 10.7448/IAS.17.1.19052.

Parkhurst, Justin and Sudeepa Abeysinghe. 2016. 'What constitutes "good" evidence for public health and social policy-making? From hierarchies to appropriateness'. *Social Epistemology* 1–15 (online version). doi: 10.1080/02691728.2016.1172365.

Pawson, Ray, Trisha Greenhalgh, Gill Harvey and Kieran Walshe. 2005. 'Realist review – a new method of systematic review designed for complex policy interventions'. *Journal of Health Services Research & Policy* 10(1): 21–34.

Pawson, Ray and Nick Tilley. 1997. *Realistic Evaluation*. London: Sage.

Payne, Geoff. 2006. 'Methodological pluralism'. In *The SAGE Dictionary of Social Research Methods*, edited by Victor Jupp, pp. 174–176. London: Sage.

Petticrew, Mark and H. Roberts. 2003. 'Evidence, hierarchies, and typologies: Horses for courses'. *Journal of Epidemiology and Community Health* 57(7): 527–529.

Rittel, Horst and Melvin Webber. 1973. 'Dilemmas in a general theory of planning'. *Policy Sciences* 4(2): 155–169.

Sanderson, Ian. 2009. 'Intelligent policy making for a complex world: pragmatism, evidence and learning'. *Political Studies* 57(4): 699–719.

Saunders, Ruth, Martin Evans and Praphul Joshi. 2005. 'Developing a process-evaluation plan for assessing health promotion program implementation: A how-to guide'. *Health Promotion Practice* 6(2): 134–147. doi: 10.1177/1524839904273387.

Seeley, Janet, Charlotte Watts, Susan Kippax, Steven Russell, Lori Heise and Alan Whiteside. 2012. 'Addressing the structural drivers of HIV: A luxury or necessity for programmes?' *Journal of the International AIDS Society* 15(Supplement 1).

Sen, Amartya. 1990. 'Development as capability expansion'. In *Human Development and the International Development Strategy for the 1990s*, edited by Keith Griffin and John Knight, pp. 41–58. London: Macmillan.

——. 1999. *Development as Freedom*. Oxford: Oxford University Press.

Shaxson, Louise. 2005. 'Is your evidence robust enough? Questions for policy makers and practitioners'. *Evidence & Policy: A Journal of Research, Debate and Practice* 1(1): 101–112. doi: 10.1332/1744264052703177.

Stone, Deborah. 2002. *Policy Paradox: The Art of Political Decision-Making*. London: W.W. Norton.

Sumartojo, E. 2000. 'Structural factors in HIV prevention: Concepts, examples, and implications for research'. *AIDS* 14(1): S3–10.

Taylor and Francis Online. 2015. '*Journal of Development Effectiveness*: Aims and scope'. http://www.tandfonline.com/action/journalInformation?show=aimsScope&journalCode=rjde20, accessed 1 July 2016.

UK Government. 2013. *What Works: Evidence Centres for Social Policy*. London: UK Cabinet Office.

Wilkinson, Richard. 2002. *Unhealthy Societies: The Afflictions of Inequality*. London: Routledge.

Worrall, John. 2010. 'Evidence: Philosophy of science meets medicine'. *Journal of Evaluation in Clinical Practice* 16(2): 356–362. doi: 10.1111/j.1365-2753.2010.01400.x.

7 What is the 'good use of evidence' for policy?

This chapter continues the discussion of what is needed to improve the use of evidence in policymaking from a political perspective by fundamentally addressing the question of what constitutes the 'good use of evidence' for policy. However, this is a question that is particularly concerned with the process through which evidence informs policy decisions, as opposed to the evidentiary content per se. Such a perspective aims to move beyond past limitations of the EBP movement discussed in Chapter 2 that has at times equated 'better' to simply mean 'more' evidence use (particularly evidence of particular types) and helps to further address many of the concerns raised by critical authors about the risk of depoliticisation of the policymaking process when evidence is invoked.

Rejecting 'good' evidence? The importance of legitimacy

Chapter 6's conceptualisation of 'good evidence for policy' helps to address some of the main concerns over both technical and issue bias explored earlier. Issue bias was particularly captured within the concept of *appropriateness* – recognising that in order for evidence to be relevant, it will need to deal with the multiple (often competing or contested) concerns of interest to policymakers. Technical bias, on the other hand, was captured through the reiteration of the importance of methodological rigour and quality, but with the important clarification that quality standards should be set by the scientific practices relevant to each form of evidence most relevant to policy needs. The chapter drew upon work by Cash et al. (2002, 2003), who identified three key features of scientific evidence that appeared important for influencing policy within a set of case studies on sustainable development: *credibility*, *salience* and *legitimacy*. Credibility and salience were expanded upon in developing the framework of what constitutes good evidence for policy. Here, however, we take up the third element – that of legitimacy.

An explicit focus on legitimacy is important because although the conceptualisation of appropriateness notes that evidence should address multiple social concerns, there are still important questions about the processes through which those concerns are elucidated, selected or ultimately acted upon. Furthermore, we can find examples where seemingly rigorous and appropriate pieces of evidence have been rejected by decision makers, not necessarily due to perceived flaws in the evidence or to a belief that the evidence speaks to the wrong policy concerns (in other words, not due to perceived technical or issue bias), but rather because the process through which the evidence was brought to bear was somehow seen to be illegitimate.

This concern is arguably particularly important in the field of international development, where there has been a long history of concern about outside influence over national policies and political agendas (Chabal 1992). Many low-income settings have been subject to historical colonial rule, but a range of authors further critique modern aid and development efforts that can appear to impose foreign ideas or agendas on countries, potentially to the detriment of state sovereignty or local decision-making processes (cf. Okuonzi and Macrae 1995; Whitfield 2009). This concern specifically speaks to the legitimacy of policy processes involved and not necessarily the final policy content.

One example of this can be seen in the resistance shown by Malawi's government to global calls to scale up provision of male circumcision as an HIV prevention intervention. From an epidemiological perspective, the procedure was identified in the mid-2000s to be an effective mechanism to reduce the spread of HIV in heterosexual epidemics, based on three independent randomised trials that each found significantly lower rates of HIV infection in circumcised compared to non-circumcised men (Mills et al. 2008). As a result, the World Health Organization and the UNAIDS programme have described male circumcision as an 'evidence-based' prevention strategy, calling for a number of African countries to scale up access to the procedure (World Health Organization and UNAIDS 2011). Yet while some countries, such as Kenya, have made significant efforts to make the procedure available, in Malawi there was a great deal of political resistance to the provision of male circumcision for HIV prevention. However, an investigation into this situation found that the resistance derived, in part, from a perception that the procedure was being demanded by international aid donors (Parkhurst, Chilongozi and Hutchinson 2015). The study describes a 'narrative of defiance' through which local politicians opposed its uptake by framing it as a case of external domination, with one official quoted as saying: 'Donors must not force male circumcision onto the Ministry . . . say do it! No, that is irresponsible science' (quoted in Parkhurst, Chilongozi and Hutchinson 2015, p. 18).

The term 'irresponsible science' is particularly relevant in this quote. The science in this case is judged irresponsible not because the evidence itself was necessarily *flawed*, but rather because of the idea that international agencies would *impose* the issue on a country. And yet this is not the only case where we can see a concern over the process through which evidence is used. Knapp and Trainor, for instance studied how climate science was used to inform decision making in the US state of Alaska, finding that while there was a need for rapid assessment of changing information: 'Information may be seen as illegitimate if the processes or the application of knowledge are seen as unfair' (2003, p. 1297). The authors further noted that stakeholders and laypersons could be concerned when the processes of using evidence was felt to exclude local knowledge or if expert scientific information was only provided in a top-down manner.

However, even amongst scientific experts who sit within specialised technical bodies, perceptions about the process of evidence utilisation may be important for the final acceptance of decisions. The World Health Organization's Global Malaria Programme, for instance, is an expert body based in Geneva that produces global guidelines for the treatment and prevention of malaria. A recent analysis of work undertaken by this body attempted to explain why the guideline development process could at times appear smooth and agreeable, while at other times it could stagnate or face opposition. The analysis found that an important element to explain this was whether the experts involved judged the guideline development process itself to be fair. For some members of this highly technical body, the *transparency* of the steps taken was critical and potentially more important than achieving consensus over the evidence itself. As one individual stated:

> There should be a way in which recommendations are made, it should be seen as open, fair, that everyone has a chance to contribute, and that their contribution will be given due weight. Not that you can always accommodate every view, you can't always get consensus, but people should say it was an open fair transparent process, even if they disagree with the conclusion.
>
> (Quoted in D'Souza 2014, p. 24)

Legitimacy in an evidence-informed policy process

These examples clearly highlight the importance of the perceived legitimacy of the process through which evidence is used to inform policy decisions. Yet the concept of political legitimacy is a broader one in the academic literature, with political scientist Fritz Scharpf, for instance, distinguishing between two key forms: *input legitimacy* and *output legitimacy*. For Scharpf, input legitimacy refers to 'trust in institutional arrangements that are thought to ensure that governing processes are generally responsive to the manifest preferences of the governed' – or 'government by the people', while output legitimacy represents 'effective solutions to common problems of the governed' – or 'government for the people' (2006, p. 1). Others have expanded on this by adding a third element, termed *throughput legitimacy* (Bekkers and Edwards 2007; Lieberherr 2013; Schmidt 2013). While input legitimacy reflects the need to have policymaking bodies that are broadly representative of the people, throughput legitimacy reflects how those bodies work in practice, which Schmidt explains captures their 'efficacy, accountability, and transparency . . . along with their inclusiveness and openness to consultation *with* the people' (2013, p. 2, emphasis in original).

Both Scharpf and Schmidt developed their ideas by writing about the European Union, specifically considering the challenges that transnational decision making can bring when responsibility for social policy is delegated to an external authority (i.e. other than the nation-state). The political scientist Robert Dahl (1994) also looked at this question of delegation to transnational bodies and coined the term 'democratic dilemma' to refer to the trade-off between what he described as 'system effectiveness' and 'democratic deliberation' that can arise in such cases. Yet in many ways, the issues involved in transnational policymaking parallels the challenges that arise when elements of social policy decision making are delegated to scientific expert bodies or technical agencies within countries as well, with a number of authors raising analogous questions about the nature of democratic representation, accountability or deliberation when policymakers defer to expert advice to inform decisions (cf. Collins and Evans 2002; Fischer 2009; Jasanoff 2011; Liberatore and Funtowicz 2003; Nowotny 2003; Weale 2001).

A number of authors reflecting on the balance between scientific expert advice and democratic principles draw on the work of Jürgen Habermas, a social theorist who is particularly known for his discussions of democracy and deliberation within the 'public space' (Habermas 1989) and who has described a continuum over which science can be seen to either dominate politics or to play a merely informative role (Habermas 1971). Scholten, for instance, reflects on Habermas' insights that the relationship between science and policy 'is often structured in such a way that the rationality of the expert dominates political decision-making and reduces value choices and goal-setting to technical and rational issues' (2011, p. 48). However, this 'technocratic model' reflects some of the core objections by critics of the EBP movement who are concerned with the depoliticisation of decision making. Hoppe similarly notes that at the end of the spectrum where technocratic ideas have primacy, 'science dominates or displaces politics', yet: 'From a democratic point of view, the technocratic stance is considered politically objectionable, if not taboo' (2005, p. 207).

Yet a concern over technocracy and its impact on democratic principles was also raised nearly a century ago by John Dewey. His widely cited work *The Public and its Problems* is particularly concerned with the idea of achieving democratic ideals, seeing governmental institutions as a means to do so (1954 [1927], p. 143). Yet Dewey recognised that reliance on experts arising from the 'technically complicated' nature of government affairs can present a key challenge to these ideals (1954 [1927], p. 124). According to Fischer, Dewey's approach to this challenge was to delineate a division of labour where 'experts would identify and analyse basic social and economic problems', while 'citizens and their political representatives would democratically set out an agenda for dealing with them' (2009, p. 5). Rogers further explains that: '[Dewey] specifically ties the idea of representative government to deliberation among the citizenry . . . he believes this will ensure that justification of one's actions remains accountable to the public . . . [and] will mitigate any blind faith we might otherwise place in political institutions' (2012, p. 4).

These discussions particularly highlight two key concepts as important to keep technocratic tendencies at bay: those of democratic *representation* and public *deliberation.* However, these elements will need to be built into what Scharpf refers to as the 'institutional arrangements', which ensure that governing processes reflect popular preferences. Yet institutional theorising in the policy sciences recognises that institutions can be thought of broadly – not just in terms of formal structures, but also the rules that shape how decisions are made, as well as the established practices (or norms) in existence that further direct outcomes (Lowndes and Roberts 2013; Peters 2005). Applied to the issue of evidence use for policymaking, then, we can use an institutional lens to discuss what can be termed the *evidence advisory system* in place, consisting of the structures, rules and norms that dictate which evidence is used, how and by whom – and we can further ask how these systems can ensure public representation and political legitimacy in the use of evidence.

Input legitimacy: constructing a legitimate evidence advisory system

Applying the three elements of political legitimacy described above, the first aspect we can consider within evidence advisory systems can be that of input legitimacy, described by Scharpf as government 'by the people', and which is particularly captured within formal system arrangements. These are important, of course, because the structures, rules and norms through which evidence is provided will fundamentally determine which bodies of evidence are considered relevant, who is given the right to speak, whether appeals can be made and a host of other factors with implications for how (or whether) the public's interests are represented in the evidence-utilisation process.

However, there are two key ways in which public representation can be considered within formal system arrangements. The first is when agents take responsibility to design the institutional features of the evidence-advisory system, while the second concerns who holds ultimate responsibility or authority for policy decisions informed by evidence. In other words, we can argue that democratic input legitimacy can be strengthened for evidence advisory systems if they are designed by an agent with a mandate to represent the population served, but also when final decision-making authority rests with representatives of the public.

Representation in the designers of evidence advisory systems

One of the biggest challenges for those aiming to improve evidence use is the fact that there is a huge array of structures that can serve to provide evidence within a policy system. Halligan (1995), for instance, discusses 'policy advisory systems' more broadly and classifies them according to two administrative features: the *location* of the advice provider in terms of whether it is internal or external to government; and the *degree of control* government has over the policy advice. He explains that three principles are central to 'good advisory systems': the provision of multiple sources of advice; flexibility to choose a mix of advisors and processes suitable to particular policy issues; and an ability to review the effectiveness of advice given. Yet Halligan also notes that there is no consensus on which structure works best to achieve these, stating that 'the verdict is still out on what structure works best for policy advice' (1995, p. 162).

However, what is critical to recognise from the perspective of input legitimacy is that someone or some group must take responsibility to choose which set of arrangements will be utilised or which responsibilities are allocated to different agencies in the first place. Yet, to build legitimacy, these decisions will most likely need to be made by a political agent with an official mandate to represent the public – undertaking what can be described as a 'stewardship' role in the shaping of these evidentiary arrangements (Alvarez-Rosette, Hawkins and Parkhurst 2013).

The idea that national administrative systems (of which evidence providing systems could be seen as a sub-set) should be constructed or shaped by representatives of the people may seem self-evident to some readers, but the colonial experience of many low-income countries can again be illustrative of instances where this has not always been the case. Indeed, the mismatch between the bureaucratic structures inherited from the colonial administration and local civil society has been hypothesised to be a key barrier to socio-economic development in these settings (Haque 1997). As such, it may not only be *policies* imposed from outside that are seen as illegitimate, but *administrative systems* that face legitimacy challenges as well (Chazan et al. 1999; Mamdani 1997).

In recent years, we have also started seeing international donor aid being spent on efforts designed to improve the use of evidence in policy in low and middle-income countries. Examples include: the Australian government's establishment of a 15-year 'knowledge support initiative' with Indonesia which aims 'to improve the quality of public policies . . . through the use of research, analysis, and evidence'(ODI 2013); the UK Department for International Development (DFID) investing £13 million in its Building Capacity to Use Research Evidence programme, which aims 'to improve development interventions through better decision making processes' (BCURE undated); and the support given by the Gates and Rockefeller Foundations to the International Decision Support Initiative, which provides training and capacity building for government bodies to increase their use of health economics tools such as cost-utility analysis for priority setting (iDSI undated). Such efforts are typically justified in terms of improving decision-making quality or effectiveness. Yet if these efforts alter the underlying administrative structures, rules or processes by which evidence informs decisions – fundamentally changing evidence advisory systems – there will be an important need to consider the implications on how interests are represented and to ask whether such institutional changes are perceived as legitimate by local populations.

However, outside of official government bureaucracies, there will obviously also be a range of independent bodies providing policy-relevant evidence to decision makers. Indeed, there can be huge numbers of think tanks, research institutes, academic bodies and civil society groups serving this role, with one review of knowledge brokers for health systems in Europe, for example, identifying 398 such bodies in an initial analysis (Lavis et al. 2013). Yet while most non-state evidence-providing bodies may be outside of direct government control, there will likely be formal and informal arrangements in place that shape when and how they inform government decision making. Again, choices will need to be made as to the exact arrangements in place, but the legitimacy of the evidence advisory system may rest on whether there is an accepted mandate in place for the agent who sets those arrangements.

Final decision authority represents the people

However, a second important element in ensuring input legitimacy from a perspective of democratic representation will be to ensure that final decision authority remains in the hands of bodies representative of, and accountable to, local populations. Within evidence advisory systems, there will obviously be a need to rely on expertise and to place some decision-making responsibility in the hands of expert bodies – to identify relevant evidence, to rank evidentiary quality or to independently provide summaries or develop guidelines, for example. Yet the tension between technocracy and democracy points to a need to ensure that scientific expertise does not replace public values in political decisions. In addition to the conceptual discussions of this tension noted above, corresponding debates have been raised across a number of empirical cases, including in discussions of food policy (Kimura 2010), monetary policy (Freeman 2002), environmental policy (Fine and Owen 2005) and pharmaceutical policy (Abraham and Sheppard 1997), amongst others.

Ensuring that final authority over social policy decisions is in the hands of public representatives can thus serve as a way to draw a line between technical expertise serving policy maker needs and technical interests replacing public values. There will, of course, be cases where technical bodies are asked to make definitive judgements in policy processes, but in such cases it may also be important to ensure there are still mechanisms by which public representatives can over-rule decisions otherwise allocated to expert bodies if those decisions are felt to be outside the public interest. One example of how this plays out in the UK is presented in Box 7.1 below.

Box 7.1 Decision authority over cancer drug provision in the UK

In the UK, the National Institute for Health Care and Excellence (NICE) serves as a semi-autonomous body with an official government mandate to undertake evidence reviews and make assessments of the affordability of treatments provided in the government-run National Health Service (NHS) (NICE 2013b). The establishment of NICE by the government in 1999 clearly reflects input legitimacy in the fact that those agents establishing the structures and rules of NICE had a mandate as part of the democratically elected government of the time. Yet of particular interest is that the agency has been granted binding decision-making authority over some elements of health service provision in parts of the UK – with the governments of England and Wales, for example, mandated to provide treatments if they have been recommended by NICE (Sorenson et al. 2008). This may at first appear to stand in contrast to the second aspect of input legitimacy discussed above, which argues that final decision-making authority should rest with representatives of the public. However, within the British political system, the legislature (Parliament) does, in fact, maintain ultimate authority as the highest power to decide how to allocate public resources and, as such, can over-ride or bypass decisions otherwise allocated to NICE.

An example of this can be seen in the case of how Parliament responded to a number of high-profile cases in which NICE recommended against providing new, costly cancer drugs on the NHS. The mechanism NICE uses for making such decisions is an assessment of cost-effectiveness (specifically cost per 'quality-adjusted life-year') (NICE 2013a, 2013a). The driving rationale for this system is one of equity, based on the idea that health impacts (premature death, illness, disability) occurring from different conditions should be valued in the same way. So, in theory, the system would spend the same amount to extend the life of a patient with renal failure as it would for one with heart disease (in otherwise equal individuals). Yet, in the UK, there appears to be particularly vocal support for cancer treatment and high levels of media attention if cancer drugs are deemed to be too expensive to justify their provision within the NHS. While the public and politicians do not necessarily believe that the calculations within the NICE decisions are flawed in these cases, there is still clearly dissatisfaction with the result of that expert body's decision-making process. As such, in 2011 the government established a special earmarked 'Cancer Drug Fund' to allocate additional government resources for cancer treatments judged to be outside the cost-effective thresholds set by NICE (UK Department of Health 2011). In this case, the democratically elected government decided to essentially bypass the rules of the legitimately established evidence advisory system, but did so in response to perceptions of public demand or changing social values (Linley and Hughes 2013). In this example, the 'social values' at stake could be seen as unfair from the perspective of some scientific experts (as it excludes people requiring more expensive treatments for non-cancer-related conditions), but retaining input legitimacy and avoiding technocracy requires structures that can allow the public to change its reasoning and its decision-making priorities, even if the legitimate expert advisory bodies disagrees.

Accepting irrationality

However, placing final decision authority in political representatives can cause particular worry to advocates of EBP who are concerned with the perceived misuse of evidence by politicians and other pubic representatives. Indeed, some might argue that the UK government example presented in Box 7.1 represents 'irrationality' on the part of the government, giving into social whims against a scientific consensus. Yet this cuts to the core of the tension between democracy and technocracy, and the recognition that democratic choices may not fit technical ideals at all times. Indeed, Mulgan has argued that: 'In a democracy, the people, and the politicians who represent them, have every right to ignore evidence' (2005, p. 224).

Nevertheless, *ignoring evidence* can take a number of meanings and it is worth unpacking this concept further. In some cases, bodies of evidence will be ignored because they have little relevance to the policy considerations at hand or they speak to policy considerations of a low priority. As such, it would be widely accepted for a government to ignore those bodies of evidence that are not appropriate to the policy consideration at hand. The example of the robust evidence on the effectiveness of *Viagra* was presented in Chapter 2 to show an obvious case where a strong evidence base might not be the most relevant to inform health planning. Indeed, in such a case, most evidence advocates would accept it if a government chose to ignore the evidence on *Viagra*'s effectiveness based on an explicit consideration of the relative importance of that piece of evidence vis-à-vis other policy goals. The shift in language some authors have made to discuss 'evidence-*informed* policymaking' (rather than 'evidence-*based* policymaking') demonstrates recognition of this dynamic (cf. Hawkins and Parkhurst 2015; Langer, Tripney and Gough 2016; Ongolo-Zogo et al. 2014). A government aware of, but dismissing, the evidence of *Viagra*'s effectiveness could be said to be making an 'informed' decision by such definitions.

Yet this logic still assumes *rationality* in decision making. 'Non-use' of evidence is accepted in this case presumably because there are other evidence bases at hand that are judged to be more relevant or because an explicit decision was made about how much priority should be given to that piece of evidence. However, the more challenging point that is raised by appeals to democratic legitimacy is that such appeals also imply that people in a democracy have the right to be *irrational* as well – that is, they have the right to simply ignore evidence altogether and make decisions for any other reasons they so choose.

A recurring frustration for advocates of evidence has unsurprisingly been when decision makers or the public select options simply because they seem to 'feel' right, regardless of, or even counter to, the indications of a body of evidence. Indeed, not only are choices at times made in democracies that ignore evidence, but according to Caplan, a result is that: 'Democracies frequently adopt and maintain policies harmful for most people' (2011, p. 1). Such situations may appear to justify a call for technocracy – the idea that people need to be protected from their own self-destructive irrationalities. Yet, as noted above, sacrificing democratic principles on an altar of technical effectiveness is widely held to be unacceptable. In many ways, this seems to imply that we must accept irrationality at times if we are to maintain key democratic principles in our uses of evidence.

That said, the cognitive sciences that were so helpful in understanding the subtle origins of political bias in Chapter 5 can also help to explain so-called irrational situations when people pursue what 'feels right' in the face of evidence. Indeed, while these cases may be frustrating from a technocratic perspective, it is actually well understood that individuals hold affinity to particular ideas – including policy choices – not because of analytical evaluations of outcomes, but because of how the construction of those ideas align with other deeply held worldviews or ideologies (Caplan 2011; Lakoff 2008; Westen 2007).

Lakoff (2002), for instance, has explored how a great deal of policy reasoning in the US is not analytical, but metaphorical, and can be traced to how well policy concepts align with one of two contrasting moral belief systems: either a 'strict father morality', which holds that people should take responsibility for themselves and that children should adhere to strict rules through discipline (so as to behave correctly in the future); or a 'nurturant parent morality', which emphasises caring for others and being cared for, with children's ideas embraced (so as to be caring in the future). Lakoff demonstrates that these moral foundations can explain many instances of potential irrationality – for example, when individuals who oppose abortion, presumably based on an argument about the sanctity of life, will also support capital punishment. 'Evidence' of the number of deaths involved obviously does not convince in this case, but rather the policy positions can be better explained by the shared moral principle they reflect – punishing wrongdoing (criminals being seen to do wrong by breaking laws and mothers of unwanted pregnancies being seen to do wrong by breaking behavioural fiats). Lakoff gives another example of the seeming rejection of an otherwise 'rational' argument in the following anecdote:

> A liberal supporter of California's 1994 single-payer [health care] initiative was speaking to a conservative audience and decided to appeal to their financial self-interest. He pointed out that the savings in administrative costs would get them the same health benefits for less money while also paying for health care for the indigent. A woman responded, 'It just sounds wrong to me. I would be paying for somebody else'.
>
> (2002, p. 25)

Again, this quote would likely frustrate many advocates of EBP, yet it reflects the reality of many political decision-making processes. Ultimately people and their representatives make decisions based on what they feel to be right rather than what experts tell them is optimal. In economics and decision science, such forms of decision making are referred to as 'irrational'. Yet the cognitive sciences drawn upon in Chapter 5 in particular have explored how human irrationality is not an exception, but rather a quite common occurrence, with Caplan (2001) going so far as to term the phenomenon 'rational irrationality' to reflect its natural origins. Understanding these mechanisms can be useful to consider how we may build evidence advisory systems to address these aspects of irrationality, or at least make them as transparent as possible in the policy process.

Output legitimacy: dealing with bias and irrationality

One way to start to address the irrationality that can arise in policy decision making is to establish norms or expectations for *output* legitimacy alongside those of *input* legitimacy. Output legitimacy fundamentally can be seen as linked to the outcomes that result from the operation of the evidence advisory system or, repeating Scharpf's definition, involving 'effective solutions to common problems of the governed' (2006, p. 1). This concern for effectiveness reminds us that evidence can indeed be a tool to achieve desired social outcomes and that robust and valid uses of evidence remain important, even if public representatives have a right to irrationality.

Achieving output legitimacy requires efforts to avoid both technical bias and issue bias as well. The former is perhaps more obvious, as the use of technically biased evidence would naturally lead to inefficient policy choices for any given goal, yet our political concern in this book recognises that the 'problems of the governed' are often multiple and competing. As such, developing 'effective solutions' for these problems will require what was discussed in the previous chapter as *good evidence for policy* – not just evidence of technical quality, but *appropriate evidence* which ensures that the high-quality evidence used is relevant to the policy concerns, is constructed in useful ways and is applicable to the local context.

So, while ensuring input legitimacy may open the door for irrational uses of evidence, working to achieve output legitimacy requires thinking about how to structure the organisations, rules and norms of evidence advisory systems to make such irrationality *less likely* and *more obvious*. Democratic societies may have a right to ignore evidence, but legitimate evidence advisory systems could make this harder to do or at least more evident when it does happen. So, for example, systems can build in the use of fact-checking structures that require decision makers to think twice about a decision that may instinctively 'feel right' – forcing them to at least look at relevant evidence they might initially have ignored. Alternatively, formal government evidence authorities may decide to publish principles of evidentiary good practice (such as what a rigorous review of evidence looks like or what a cherry-picked review looks like) that can serve as clear templates to judge whether policy decisions are taken in contradiction to scientific principles – effectively allowing public scrutiny over political uses of evidence with reference to an established scientific authority. The following chapter will explore other examples of institutional structures or rules that can address forms of evidentiary bias, but what is critical here is to recognise that while input legitimacy may require final decision authority to rest in the hands of public representatives, output legitimacy enables reflection on how to actively design systems to mitigate instances of irrationality.

Throughput legitimacy: representation as evidence is being used

The final element of legitimacy to consider within systems of evidence advice is that of throughput legitimacy, which can be seen as focused on the actual functioning of advisory systems. Throughput legitimacy is important because even if final decision-making authority lies in public representatives (as part of input legitimacy), there can still be legitimacy challenges if technical considerations utilised throughout the process of evidence identification, review and provision do not perfectly align with the goals or values of the public.

In an editorial in the journal *Evidence & Policy*, for instance, Boaz, Locock and Ward (2015) lament the absence of direct representation of people affected by the evidence used to inform policy. They ask: 'isn't the point of acquiring all this knowledge, and mobilising it, to make things better for people on the receiving end? Where is their voice in what knowledge is mobilised and how?' The authors further note that 'it is . . . possible that researchers make unfounded assumptions about what matters to the public and users, and seek to mobilise knowledge which is marginal to their interests' (2015, p. 147). Similarly, Sanderson (2009) is critical of how the modern EBP discourse removes political realities from the policy sphere, arguing that what is needed instead is a dynamic system of 'policy learning' that is fundamentally based on processes of deliberation in the form of channels of communication between government and civil society.

However, reliance on deliberation to provide political legitimacy is a key principle within a broader body of work on the concept of 'deliberative democracy' in the academic literature. Writing on this subject, Fishkin and Luskin define deliberation as 'a weighing of competing considerations' and explain that it is achieved through discussions that have particular characteristics, including a need to be *informed* by 'accurate factual claims' and that need to be *comprehensive* in terms of giving attention to 'all points of view held by significant proportions of the population' (2005, p. 40). Cohen has further stated that 'outcomes are democratically legitimate if and only if they could be the object of a free and reasoned agreement among equals' (2003, p. xv), while Weale notes that the work of Habermas provides a theoretical foundation for the importance of deliberation in democracy, seeing 'the legitimacy of a legal system as depending upon the engagement of citizens communicating with one another' (2007, p. 79).

Some have seen the need for deliberation (and deliberative democratic principles) as particularly important when public policy relies on delegation to outside agencies, including expert bodies providing scientific advice (cf. Gutmann and Thompson 2009; van Eeten 2001). Authors in the field of science and technology studies (STS) in particular have considered these issues by investigating how the science–policy interface works to integrate public interests, values or needs through a dynamic and ongoing process that delineates what constitutes policy-relevant science and expertise (Gieryn 1999; Hoppe 2005; Jasanoff 1987, 1996).

So, for example, Liberatore and Funtowicz have argued that the 'democratisation of expertise' requires *transparency* through 'processes enabling the "tracking" of how decisions are made, by whom, on what basis' (2003, p. 147) (see also Jasanoff 2006). *Public participation* and *deliberation,* on the other hand, are widely promoted to resist the 'scientization' of politics (De Jong and Mentzel 2001; Fischer 2003; Habermas 1971; Wynne 2007). Jasanoff, for instance, has pointed to an instrumental need to consider the practices of governance that best serve to solicit public input in matters to do with science and technology, although she warns against simply 'placating citizens with rituals of participation' (2011, p. 624). Rayner (2003) further explains that public participation in the form of community advisory bodies, consensus conferences and other such arrangements have particularly emerged to increase representation to the public in an era of electoral (voting) decline (but he notes that there has not yet been sufficient evaluation of their impact).

A need for more direct deliberation with the public in the process of evidence use was also seen in the empirical work of Cash et al. (2003), whose initial framework provided a springboard for much of the discussion in this and the previous chapter. In their analysis of the use of science and technology to inform sustainable development planning, for instance, they found that:

> [Knowledge systems] that made a serious commitment to managing boundaries between expertise and decision making more effectively linked knowledge to action than those that did not. Such systems invested in *communication, translation, and/or mediation* and, thereby, more effectively balanced salience, credibility, and legitimacy in the information they produced.
> (2003, p. 8089, emphasis added)

Efforts of these kinds – active communication, public consultation and participation, and transparency throughout the evidence-utilisation process – can be seen as contributing to throughput legitimacy. Ultimately, just as there are no right or wrong answers about how to build the structures that govern the evidence advisory system, there is equally no single answer to the question of how to structure deliberation into the processes of evidence utilisation or how much deliberation is required per se. Rather, the goal here has been to identify the principles that can guide decisions in these areas, which will ultimately be taken up to different extents and in different forms, depending on the local political culture and context.

Discussion: a legitimacy framework for the good use of evidence

There can be obvious tensions between a desire to achieve the best possible social goals from a body of evidence and respect for a democratic decision-making process. This tension cuts to the core of the question of what constitutes the 'good use of evidence' when a desire to avoid technical bias and maximise the potential of evidence to achieve social goals risks depoliticisation and a trend towards technocracy. As discussed in the introductory chapters, the approach taken in this book has been to recognise the importance and validity of both sets of normative concerns in our thinking about how to improve the use of evidence in policymaking. That said, at times trade-offs will exist or a balance will need to be struck between conflicting ideas within local decision-making contexts. This chapter has explained that many aspects of this balance will be shaped by the institutional features making up local *evidence advisory systems* – systems of structures, rules and norms that will direct how evidence is used within policymaking.

The good use of evidence for policymaking ultimately reflects judgements on the legitimacy of the establishment and operation of evidence advisory systems, with three key aspects of legitimacy – input, output and throughput – being used to explore these ideas. The discussion in the previous chapter of 'good evidence for policy' covered the need to ensure the utilisation of *high-quality* evidence that is *appropriate* to policy needs. This was shown to capture much of the idea of output legitimacy as it is commonly understood. But the exploration of input and throughput legitimacy further highlighted the central importance of democratic principles within the construction and operation of decision-making systems.

Input legitimacy was captured by ensuring that evidence advisory systems themselves are developed by those groups who hold some official public *mandate* (with government officials typically taking a *stewardship* role) and by ensuring that final policy decision *authority* lies with public representatives. Throughput legitimacy, on the other hand, was seen to capture aspects of legitimacy arising from the operation of those systems in practice. Drawing on scholars of deliberative democracy and STS, the importance of *transparency* and *public deliberation* was particularly promoted due to a need to have a public check in place over systems that delegate some forms of decision authority to outside expert bodies.

Taken in combination, these ideas can construct a 'legitimacy framework' for evidence-informed policy processes, presented in Table 7.1 below.

Table 7.1 Legitimacy framework for evidence-informed policy processes

Legitimacy dimension	*Concerned with*	*Represented in*	*Achieved via*
Input	Democratic representation within the system.	**Structures** of the evidence advisory system (EAS): • formal structures – evidence advisory bodies; • established rules – which evidence is consulted, when and how; • norms of practice – de facto rules and functions.	**Stewardship**: structures developed by a *stewardship* body with a popular *mandate* to establish the institutional form of the EAS. **Authority**: final decision-making *authority* lies with democratically representative bodies.
Throughput	Democratic deliberation in the operation of the system.	**Operational processes**: the process and the functioning of the EAS, e.g.: • the choice of evidence; • the application of evidence; • the process through which evidence is used within the EAS.	**Deliberation** • active communication; • public consultation/engagement; • advisory bodies; • transparency rules; • appeals processes.

(continued)

Table 7.1 (continued)

Legitimacy dimension	*Concerned with*	*Represented in*	*Achieved via*
Output	Scientific fidelity in operation and outcomes (avoiding technical and issue bias).	**Outcomes**: the resultant use of *good evidence for policy* – captured by *appropriateness*: • evidence relevant to those policy concerns; • evidence constructed in ways useful in relation to decision-makers' goals; • evidence applicable to the local policy context.	**Goal clarification** • explicit identification of policy concerns; • critical reflection on evidentiary needs in reference to policy goals. **Applying quality criteria for multiple forms of evidence**: • unbiased; • methodologically rigorous; • systematic. **Reducing bias** or **making bias more evident**: structures and rules that make technical bias, issue bias and irrationality less likely, more evident and/or open to scrutiny.

The political perspective drawn upon throughout this book has provided a range of insights into how evidence use for policymaking is fundamentally different from evidence use from a purely technical perspective. If we accept the premises that (a) policymaking involves choices between competing interests and trade-offs amongst social values, (b) political decision-making processes are structured within institutional arrangements, and (c) political processes require legitimacy to be accepted, then we can apply the frameworks developed so far to address many of the overlapping normative concerns at stake in the use of evidence to inform policy. Rather than simply working to increase scientific communication or the 'uptake' of research findings, improving the use of evidence for policymaking can be seen as involving the establishment of formal evidence advisory systems, designed by a legitimate representative body, which serves to reduce both technical and issue bias in the evidence utilised. It also requires decision authority to rest in the hands of those who are representative of, and accountable to, local populations, and processes to be in place that produce some form of transparency and deliberation with the public. However, taken in combination, these principles reflect a set of normative concerns that can establish an overarching concept of the *good governance of evidence* – to which the next and final chapter will now turn.

References

Abraham, John and Julie Sheppard. 1997. 'Democracy, technocracy, and the secret state of medicines control: Expert and nonexpert perspectives'. *Science, Technology & Human Values* 22(2): 139–167.

Alvarez-Rosette, Arturo, Ben Hawkins and Justin Parkhurst. 2013. *Health System Stewardship and Evidence Informed Health Policy*. London: GRIP-Health Programme, London School of Hygiene and Tropical Medicine.

BCURE. undated. 'Building capacity to use research evidence: BCURE'. https://bcure global.wordpress.com, accessed 6 July 2016.

Bekkers, Victor and Arthur Edwards. 2007. 'Legitimacy and democracy: A conceptual framework for assessing governance practices'. In *Governance and the Democratic Deficit: Assessing the Democratic Legitimacy of Governance Practices*, edited by Victor Bekkers, Geske Dijkstra, Arthur Edwards and Menno Fenger, pp. 35–60. Aldershot: Ashgate.

Boaz, Annette, Louise Locock and Vicky Ward. 2015. 'Whose evidence is it anyway?' *Evidence & Policy* 11(2): 145–148.

Caplan, Bryan. 2001. 'Rational ignorance versus rational irrationality'. *Kyklos* 54(1): 3–26.

——. 2011. *The Myth of the Rational Voter: Why Democracies Choose Bad policies.* Princeton: Princeton University Press.

Cash, David, William Clark, Frank Alcock, Nancy Dickson, Noelle Eckley and Jill Jäger. 2002. *Salience, Credibility, Legitimacy and Boundaries: Linking Research, Assessment and Decision Making.* Cambridge, MA: John F. Kennedy School of Government, Harvard University.

Cash, David, William Clark, Frank Alcock, Nancy Dickson, Noelle Eckley, David Guston, Jill Jäger and Ronald B Mitchell. 2003. 'Knowledge systems for sustainable development'. *Proceedings of the National Academy of Sciences* 100(14): 8086–8091.

Chabal, Patrick. 1992. *Power in Africa*. London: Macmillian.

Chazan, Naomi, Peter Lewis, Robert Mortimer, Donald Rothchild and Stephen John Stedman. 1999. *Politics and Society in Contemporary Africa*, 3rd edn. Boulder: Lynne Rienner.

Cohen, Joshua. 2003. Deliberation and democratic legitimacy. In *Debates in Contemporary Political Philosophy: An Anthology*, Derek Matravers and Jon Pike, pp. 342–360. London: Routledge.

Collins, H. M. and Robert Evans. 2002. 'The third wave of science studies: Studies of expertise and experience'. *Social Studies of Science* 32(2): 235–296. doi: 10.1177/0306312702032002003.

D'Souza, Bianca. 2014. 'Strengthening policy setting processes at the World Health Organization Global Malaria Programme'. DrPH Organisational and Policy Analysis Report, Department of Global Health and Development, London School of Hygiene and Tropical Medicine.

Dahl, Robert A. 1994. 'A democratic dilemma: System effectiveness versus citizen participation'. *Political Science Quarterly* 109(1): 23–34. doi: 10.2307/2151659.

De Jong, Martin and Maarten Mentzel. 2001. 'Policy and science: Options for democratisation in European countries'. *Science and Public Policy* 28(6): 403–412. doi: 10.3152/147154301781781228.

Dewey, John. 1954 [1927]. *The Public and its Problems*. Athens, OH: Swallow Press/Ohio University Press.

Fine, James and Dave Owen. 2005. 'Technocracy and democracy: Conflicts between models and participation in environmental law and planning'. *Hastings Law Journal* 56(5): 901–982.

Fischer, Frank. 2003. *Reframing Public Policy*. Oxford: Oxford University Press.

——. 2009. *Democracy and Expertise: Reorienting Policy Inquiry*. Oxford: Oxford University Press.

Fishkin, James and Robert Luskin. 2005. 'Experimenting with a democratic ideal: Deliberative polling and public opinion'. *Acta Politica* 40(3): 284–298.

Freeman, John. 2002. 'Competing commitments: Technocracy and democracy in the design of monetary institutions'. *International Organization* 56(4): 889–910. doi:10.1162/002081802760403810.

Gieryn, Thomas. 1999. *Cultural Boundaries of Science: Credibility on the Line*. Chicago: University of Chicago Press.

Gutmann, Amy and Dennis Thompson. 2009. *Why Deliberative Democracy?* Princeton: Princeton University Press.

Habermas, Jürgen. 1971. *Toward a Rational Society: Student Protest, Science, and Politics*. Boston: Beacon Press.

——. 1989. *The Structural Transformation of the Public Sphere: An Inquiry into a Category of Bourgeois Society*. London: Polity.

Halligan, John. 1995. 'Policy advice and the public service'. In *Governance in a Changing Environment*, edited by Guy Peters and Donald Savoie, pp. 138–172. Montreal: Canadian Centre for Management Development.

Haque, M. Shamsul. 1997. 'Incongruity between bureaucracy and society in developing nations: A critique'. *Peace & Change* 22(4): 432–462. doi: 10.1111/0149-0508.00061.

Hawkins, Benjamin and Justin Parkhurst. 2015. 'The "good governance" of evidence in health policy'. *Evidence & Policy: A Journal of Research, Debate and Practice*. doi: 10.1332/174426415X14430058455412.

Hoppe, Robert. 2005. 'Rethinking the science-policy nexus: From knowledge utilization and science technology studies to types of boundary arrangements'. *Poiesis & Praxis* 3(3): 199–215.

iDSI. undated. 'About us'. http://www.idsihealth.org/about-us, accessed 6 July 2016.

Jasanoff, Sheila 1987. 'Contested boundaries in policy-relevant science'. *Social Studies of Science* 17(2): 195–230.

——. 1996. 'Beyond epistemology: Relativism and engagement in the politics of science'. *Social Studies of Science* 26(2): 393–418. doi: 10.1177/030631296026002008.

——. 2006. 'Transparency in public science: Purposes, reasons, limits'. *Law and Contemporary Problems* 21–45.

——. 2011. 'Constitutional moments in governing science and technology'. *Science & Engineering Ethics* 17(4): 621–638. doi: 10.1007/s11948-011-9302-2.

Kimura, Aya Hirata. 2010. 'Between technocracy and democracy: An experimental approach to certification of food products by Japanese consumer cooperative women'. *Journal of Rural Studies* 26(2): 130–140. doi: http://dx.doi.org/10.1016/j.jrurstud.2009.09.007.

Knapp, Corrine Noel and Sarah F. Trainor. 2013. 'Adapting science to a warming world'. *Global Environmental Change* 23(5): 1296–1306. doi: http://dx.doi.org/10.1016/j.gloenvcha.2013.07.007.

Lakoff, George. 2002. *Moral Politics*, 2nd edn. Chicago: University of Chicago Press.

——. 2008. *The Political Mind: Why You Can't Understand 21st-Century Politics with an 18th-Century Brain*. New York: Viking.

Langer, Laurenz, Janice Tripney and David Gough. 2016. *The Science of Using Science: Researching the Use of Research Evidence in Decision-Making*. London: EPPI-Centre, Social Science Research Unit, UCL Institution of Education, University College London.

Lavis, John, Govin Permanand, Cristina Catallo and BRIDGE Study Team. 2013. *How Can Knowledge Brokering Be Advanced in a Country's Health System?* Copenhagen: WHO Regional Office for Europe.

Liberatore, Angela and Silvio Funtowicz. 2003. '"Democratising" expertise, "expertising" democracy: What does this mean, and why bother?' *Science and Public Policy* 30(3): 146–150. doi: 10.3152/147154303781780551.

Lieberherr, Eva. 2013. 'The role of throughput in the input output legitimacy debate: Insights from public and private governance modes in the Swiss and English water sectors'. International Conference on Public Policy, Grenoble, 26–28 June 2013.

Linley, Warren and Dyfrig Hughes. 2013. 'Societal views on NICE, cancer drugs fund and value-based pricing criteria for prioritising medicines : A cross-sectional survey of 4118 adults in Great Britain'. *Health Economics* 22(8): 948–964.

Lowndes, Vivien and Mark Roberts. 2013. *Why Institutions Matter*. Basingstoke: Palgrave Macmillan.

Mamdani, Mahmood. 1997. *Citizen and Subject: Decentralised Despotism and the Legacy of Late Colonialism*. Delhi: Oxford University Press.

Mills, E., C. Cooper, A. Anema and G. Guyatt. 2008. 'Male circumcision for the prevention of heterosexually acquired HIV infection: A meta-analysis of randomized trials involving 11,050 men'. *HIV Medicine* 9(6): 332–335. doi: 10.1111/j.1468-1293.2008.00596.x.

Mulgan, Geoff. 2005. 'Government, knowledge and the business of policymaking: The potential and limits of evidence-based policy'. *Evidence & Policy: A Journal of Research, Debate and Practice* 1(2): 215–226. doi: 10.1332/1744264053730789.

NICE. 2013a. *Guide to the Methods of Technology Appraisal 2013*. London: National Institute of Health and Care Excellence.

——. 2013b. *NICE Charter*. London: National Institute for Health and Care Excellence.

Nowotny, Helga. 2003. 'Democratising expertise and socially robust knowledge'. *Science and Public Policy* 30(3): 151–156. doi: 10.3152/147154303781780461.

ODI. 2013. 'Australia-Indonesia partnership for pro-poor policy: The knowledge sector initiative', http://www.odi.org/projects/2677-australia-indonesia-partnership-pro-poor-policy-knowledge-sector-initiative, accessed 6 July 2016.

Okuonzi, Sam Agatre and Joanna Macrae. 1995. 'Whose policy is it anyway? International and national influences on health policy development in Uganda'. *Health Policy and Planning* 10(2): 122–132.

Ongolo-Zogo, Pierre, John Lavis, Goran Tomson and Nelson Sewankambo. 2014. 'Initiatives supporting evidence informed health system policymaking in Cameroon and Uganda: A comparative historical case study'. *BMC Health Services Research* 14(1): 612. doi: 10.1186/s12913-014-0612-3.

Parkhurst, Justin, David Chilongozi and Eleanor Hutchinson. 2015. 'Doubt, defiance, and identity: Understanding resistance to male circumcision for HIV prevention in Malawi'. *Social Science & Medicine* 135: 15–22.

Peters, Guy. 2005. *Institutional Theory in Political Science*. London: Continuum.

Rayner, Steve. 2003. 'Democracy in the age of assessment: Reflections on the roles of expertise and democracy in public-sector decision making'. *Science and Public Policy* 30(3): 163–170. doi: 10.3152/147154303781780533.

Rogers, Melvin. 2012. 'Introduction'. In *The Public and its Problems*, edited by Melvin Rogers and John Dewey, pp. 1–29. University Park, PN: Penn State Press.

Sanderson, Ian. 2009. 'Intelligent policy making for a complex world: pragmatism, evidence and learning'. *Political Studies* 57(4): 699–719.

Scharpf, Fritz. 2006. *Problem-Solving Effectiveness and Democratic Accountability in the EU*. Vienna: Institute for Advanced Studies.

Schmidt, Vivien. 2013. 'Democracy and legitimacy in the European Union revisited: Input, output and "throughput"'. *Political Studies* 61(1): 2–22. doi: 10.1111/j.1467-9248.2012.00962.x.

Scholten, Peter. 2011. *Framing Immigrant Integration: Dutch Research-Policy Dialogues in Comparative Perspective.* Amsterdam: Amsterdam University Press.

Sorenson, Corinna, Michael Drummond, Panos Kanavos and Alistair McGuire. 2008. *National Institute for Health and Clinical Excellence (NICE). How Does it Work and What are the Implications for the US?* Washington DC: National Pharmaceutical Council.

UK Department of Health. 2011. *Equity and Excellence: Liberating the NHS.* London: The Stationery Office.

Van Eeten, Michel. 2001. 'The challenge ahead for deliberative democracy: In reply to Weale'. *Science and Public Policy* 28(6): 423–426. doi: 10.3152/147154301781781200.

Weale, Albert. 2001. 'Science advice, democratic responsiveness and public policy'. *Science and Public Policy* 28(6): 413–421. doi: 10.3152/147154301781781237.

——. 2007. *Democracy*. Basingstoke: Palgrave Macmilian.

Westen, Drew. 2007. *The Political Brain: The Role of Emotion in Deciding the Fate of the Nation.* New York: Public Affairs.

Whitfield, Lindsay. 2009. 'Introduction: aid and sovereignty'. In *The Politics of Aid: African Strategies for Dealing with Donors*, edited by Lindsay Whitfield, pp. 1–26. Oxford: Oxford University Press.

World Health Organization and UNAIDS. 2011. *Joint Strategic Action Framework to Accelerate the Scale-up of Voluntary Medical Male Circumcision for HIV Prevention in Eastern and Southern Africa.* Geneva: UNAIDS.

Wynne, Brian. 2007. 'Public participation in science and technology: Performing and obscuring a political-conceptual category mistake'. *East Asian Science, Technology and Society* 1(1): 99–110. doi: 10.1215/s12280-007-9004-7.

8 From evidence-based policy to the good governance of evidence

Building institutions to improve evidence use

Chapter 2 laid out a number of limitations with many current efforts to promote evidence use in policymaking. These served as springboards for subsequent chapter discussions, including the need to address the political sources of evidentiary bias, the need to consider good evidence from a policy perspective and the need to consider political legitimacy in the process of evidence utilisation. A final challenge identified in that chapter was captured in the recognition that the vast majority of work discussing how to improve evidence focuses on individuals – exploring strategies such as linking researchers and policymakers, bringing evidence to decision makers or training individuals to broker knowledge. It was noted that such efforts place undue expectations on researchers, who may not see it as their role or skill set to transfer knowledge. Furthermore, a focus on individuals also risks having limited potential to engender long-term or system-wide change, as individuals naturally leave their positions or change roles over time. This individualistic focus has led Nutley, Walter and Bland to argue that insufficient attention has been paid to the institutional arrangements that connect evidence to policy, defining institutions as 'the formal organisations established to connect evidence and policy, particularly focusing on their roles, structures, and modes of operation' (2002, p. 78). The authors further argue that this lack of attention to institutions serves as one of the main explanations for the lack of utilisation of social research in policymaking.

In political science, there has been a much deeper engagement with the concept of institutions, even if it has had limited application within the EBP field to date. The early years of the discipline have been described as particularly institutionally oriented, with a great deal of scholarship analysing the differences and functions of the organisational arrangements of government bodies (Lowndes and Roberts 2013; Peters 2005). However, newer institutional approaches within political science have particularly linked institutional analysis to questions of how social values influence policy choices, including consideration of the roles that institutions play in both shaping and embedding values and arrangements of political power (March and Olsen 1984; Peters 2005). In these ways, attention has been paid to the ways in which institutions affect democratic representation and collective decision making in particular. March and Olsen (2006) explain:

> Democratic political life is ordered by institutions . . . An institution is a relatively stable collection of rules and practices, embedded in structures of *resources* that make action possible – organizational, financial and staff capabilities, and structures of *meaning* that explain and justify behaviour – roles, identities and belongings, common purposes, and casual and normative beliefs.
>
> (2006, p. 691, emphasis in original)

Lowndes and Roberts (2013) further explain that institutions in modern conceptualisations are understood as more than just the physical structures or organisational bodies within a system, but are also captured in the rules by which such bodies operate, the practices they undertake in their operation and the discursive narratives by which their work is understood.

These insights allow us to consider two key ways that institutional change, or processes of institutionalisation, can work to shape the use of evidence in policymaking. First, this can involve building or altering the actual structures in place that are involved in evidence utilisation (including the resources and arrangements of what were termed 'evidence advisory systems' in the previous chapter). Second, they can involve changes to the principles by which those institutions operate – with principles particularly reflected by, and embedded within, the rules, incentives or practices through which institutions operate.

Government institutions: evidence advisory systems

For many, the first place to look for building institutions that influence the use of evidence for policy will be within the mechanisms of government decision making itself. Halligan (1995) has noted that there are, in fact, a very large number of structures and arrangements that can make up government advisory systems, presenting one framework that classifies advisory bodies based on their location (within the public service, internal to government or external) and the level of governmental control over their activities. Similarly, the World Health Organization's Alliance for Health Policy and Systems Research has developed a framework of 'embeddedness' to reflect the strength of the institutional arrangements that provide research evidence to health policymakers. This framework describes the location of evidentiary advice as lying in a series of concentric circles around the government – with 'government organisations' (such as official research institutions and advisory bodies) being most central, followed by 'government-supported organisations' (think tanks, consultants, sponsored academics, etc.) and finally 'independent organisations' (e.g. non-government organisations, international donors and independent academics) being most distant. In addition, however, the framework also sees embeddedness as reflecting some measure of the depth and strength of links, captured by four factors in particular: the quality of connections, the quantity of connections, agency capacity and the reputation of the evidence provider (Koon et al. 2013; Koon, Nambiar, and Rao 2012).

The concept of *stewardship* over the evidence advisory system discussed in the previous chapter pointed to a need for officials with a formal mandate to take responsibility for designing or altering evidence advisory arrangements to achieve input legitimacy. Yet, clearly, governments may officially authorise evidence to be provided in a large number of ways. Undertaking changes to improve evidence advisory systems will most likely require some critical reflection, then, on where pieces of evidence advice can enter the system and how strong or well integrated those evidence advisory structures should be.

Some ministries may wish to keep these roles within the bureaucracy, establishing their own offices of policy advice and employing technical advisors tasked with gathering or synthesising evidence. These strategies may provide the most direct and well-integrated channels for evidentiary advice, yet such bodies face capacity challenges in resource constrained settings, limiting the scope of issues for which they can actually function. Delegating evidence advice to non-government or semi-autonomous bodies can therefore be a practical strategy to increase capacity, but there are numerous other reasons why evidence advice may be delegated to outside bodies as well, including a perceived need for independence or a desire to draw on different forms of expertise outside the bureaucracy.

Many governments convene meetings of expert panels or 'technical working groups', for instance, to inform specific decisions, granting such groups varying levels of autonomy (Fouilleux, Maillard and Smith 2005; Gornitzka and Sverdrup 2008). Similarly, positions such as 'Chief Scientific Advisor' have been embedded within some government agencies to provide a formally recognised role for an expert providing a scientific perspective on government policy processes. However, the independence of roles such as these may be critical in determining how they work and if their use can address evidentiary bias. For example, the chief medical officer appointed to the UK Ministry of Health has publicly criticised the government's provision of homeopathy on the National Health Service (Silverman 2013). This independent critical voice stands in contrast to reports about the US Surgeon General in the past. According to Duncan (2007), during the George W. Bush administration, the Surgeon General was directed not to mention evidence contrary to government policy, to mention the President three times per page in every other speech and to speak in support of Republican political candidates. Such practices clearly challenge the ability for such an appointment to provide independent policy advice on technical issues.

Particular attention in recent years has also focused on the establishment of formal agencies with an official mandate to provide or synthesise evidence for policy. In the health sector, one of the most widely cited examples of this is the UK's National Institute for Health and Care Excellence (NICE) (mentioned in Chapter 7), which provides clinical guidelines, evidence summaries and technology appraisals to inform decision making and resource allocation for the National Health Service (NICE 2013; Sorenson et al. 2008). However, NICE's role in rationalising the use of evidence has been so well regarded nationally that it has served as a key model for the development of a series of 'what works' centres in other areas of UK public policymaking (UK Government 2013) and has been described as a 'national treasure' by one commentator (Godlee 2009). NICE has also been emulated in other countries. One example of this has been the establishment of Colombia's Instituto de Evaluación Tecnológica en Salud (IETS), which was designed specifically to emulate NICE by undertaking similar activities (NICE International 2011).

In the education sector, a similar example would be the Norwegian government's establishment of the Knowledge Centre for Education, which is tasked 'to produce, gather, synthesise and disseminate knowledge from research on issues of relevance to the education sector'. The Centre states that it 'adheres to internationally recognised standards on how to synthesise research on education, and to show how research can be practically applied by practitioners and policy-makers' (Knowledge Centre for Education 2015).

Establishing practices to mitigate bias

However, in addition to establishing formal structures, institutional change importantly involves establishing rules and norms that direct practices as well. All of the institutional bodies noted above will have their own working arrangements, but it is of further interest to identify cases where governments have created procedures, rules or even laws that serve to reduce bias or improve scientific good practice. Indeed, by embedding good practice in such ways, we can consider how systems may evolve such that their ongoing or continuous operational processes increasingly reflect principles of improved evidence utilisation. One well-regarded example of this is Mexico's 2004 Social Development Law, which requires new social development policies and interventions to be formally monitored and evaluated. A World Bank report described this law as representing the 'institutionalisation of evaluation' (Castro et al. 2009), establishing an expectation of good practice to generate evidence on the effects of social interventions, with the law further establishing an autonomous National Council for the Evaluation of Social Development Policy (CONEVAL) to undertake such evaluations (Lopez 2012). Another more common example of government legislation that may address sources of bias comes in the form of freedom of information legislation. While freedom of information laws obviously work to improve the transparency of governance processes, they also allow direct scrutiny of decision making and allow civil society or the media to challenge cases where evidence appears to be being misused or where decision making can be shown to be based on a selective body of evidence.

Outside of passing laws, governments may also institutionalise internal rules and procedures that serve to address sources of bias. So, for example, there can be expectations that planners follow processes akin to multi-criteria decision analysis, a decision-making approach that requires explicitly listing the multiple issues of relevance to a decision in order to assign them relative weight or priority

(Baltussen and Niessen 2006; Belton and Stewart 2002). Institutionalising such steps can help to address issue bias by effectively mandating 'goal clarification', thereby making it clear which bodies of evidence would be considered relevant to a decision. Governments can also institutionalise deliberative practices that invite multiple stakeholders to speak on issues and present arguments to technical committees, with such deliberation serving to ensure that technical agencies do not lose sight of the multiple issues relevant to a decision. Again, the UK's NICE provides a useful example. While that agency evaluates clinical treatments on the basis of cost-effectiveness, it also undertakes public consultations to identify other relevant social values to assist decision making. One result of this has been an 'end of life care' premium that the agency applies based on stakeholder demands – essentially using a higher cost-effectiveness threshold to judge the affordability of treatments which can extend life for someone with less than two years to live (Cookson 2013).

Another example of procedural efforts to overcome technical bias can be seen in the forms of 'alternative analysis' that have developed in the field of military and intelligence planning and that specifically work to address cognitive errors that can lead to premature conclusions or incorrect factual assessments. Fishbein and Treverton explain:

> Traditional intelligence analysis generates forecasts or explanations based on logical processing of available evidence, whereas alternative analysis seeks to help analysts and policy-makers stretch their thinking through structured techniques that challenge underlying assumptions and broaden the range of possible outcomes considered. Properly applied, it serves as a hedge against the natural tendencies of analysts – like all human beings – to perceive information selectively through the lens of preconceptions, to search too narrowly for facts that would confirm rather than discredit existing hypotheses, and to be unduly influenced by premature consensus within analytic groups close at hand.
>
> (2004, p. 1)

The authors list approaches such as 'divergent thinking exercises', structured dialogues to consider alternative possibilities, or undertaking simulations to help understand uncertainty in planning decisions. Establishing rules or norms that expect planners to explicitly question their potential unconscious errors can therefore be yet another way to institutionalise change that serves to address the biases arising from the politics of evidence.

Non-state institutions: experts and broader civil society

However, there are a number of other institutions outside government that also play important roles in shaping how evidence is either provided to, or utilised by, policymakers. Professional associations of scientists and national academies, academic bodies, civil society organisations and the media can all make up a broader institutional landscape influencing evidence use, and many of these can work in ways that serve to reduce or counter various forms of evidentiary bias.

National academies of science represent one such important structure in a number of countries. Typically, these aim to be independent collectives of scientists that can provide advice, guidance or norms of best practice from a scientific perspective and that can similarly serve as a critical voice against the misuse of evidence in policy debates. The US National Academies of Sciences, for example, has published informational materials that aim to provide scientific consensus on major policy areas such as stem cells, energy, transportation and drinking water, amongst others (National Academies of Sciences 2016). In another case, in order to respond to the political debates over climate change, a collective consensus statement was developed by a set of 11 such national academies (from Brazil, Canada, China, France, Germany, India, Italy, Japan, Russia, the UK and the US), stating outright their position that 'climate change is real' (Joint Academies of Science undated). Such efforts are aimed to serve as a bulwark against forms of bias such as cherry-picking or selective uses of evidence, or indeed outright denial of science as well.

Expert collectives can also serve as evidence providers and synthesising bodies to help promote more systematic uses of evidence. The Cochrane Collaboration in health care has already been mentioned and stands out as a global expert body that has established a set of best practices on systematic reviews of data, as well as serving as a repository of evidence to guide health practice (Starr et al. 2009). At times, universities can also take on evidence synthesising roles. For example, in the UK, the Evidence for Policy and Practice Information and Co-ordinating Centre (EPPI-Centre) at University College London's Institute of Education undertakes systematic reviews on policy-relevant topics related to education, health, social welfare and international development, while also providing guidance, teaching and publications on how to undertake such reviews (EPPI-Centre undated). In Uganda, alternatively, the Makerere University College of Health Sciences has developed a 'rapid response service' that can quickly synthesise evidence to inform pressing health policy decisions (Makerere University College of Health Sciences undated), while in Canada, the McMaster Health Forum serves multiple roles: as an evidence repository (i.e. hosting www.healthsystemsevidence.org), as an evidence synthesising hub and as a forum for collective problem solving (McMaster Health Forum undated).

In addition to these examples of bodies synthesising evidence, stand-alone efforts have also been established to counter specific forms of evidentiary bias that are seen to be widespread and/or problematic. One example of this is the COMPare programme at Oxford University's Centre for Evidence-Based Medicine, which was set up to address 'outcome switching' in clinical trials (discussed in Chapter 3). The project reviews previously published trials to identify cases of switched outcomes and flags these up to journal editors. The website for the programme notes what proportion of its included trials 'perfectly' reported all their pre-specified outcomes (less than 15 per cent of cases at the time of writing) and notes other key measures of bias, such as how many outcomes were 'silently added' (COMPare 2016). There are also academic efforts to promote public deliberation, such as at Stanford University (Center for Deliberative Democracy undated) or Carnegie Mellon University (Program for Deliberative Democracy 2005), which can be seen as providing resources that can potentially address issue bias when deliberative strategies work to ensure that multiple relevant social concerns are considered in evidence-informed policy decisions.

Think tanks and similar organisations also clearly play knowledge brokering roles (cf. Lavis et al. 2013; Mendizabal and Sample 2009; Smith 1991; van Kammen, de Savigny and Sewankambo 2006), although their independence may prove an important consideration in affecting whether they reflect or counter one or more forms of bias. In order to reduce issue bias in particular, it may be particularly important to identify those think tanks that take a non-partisan approach in providing policy-relevant evidence. The Pew Research Center in the US provides one example, stating that it aims not to take political positions and describes itself as 'a nonpartisan fact tank that informs the public about the issues, attitudes and trends shaping America and the world (Pew Research Center 2016).

A final sector that plays an important role in the broader institutional landscape influencing evidence use is that of the media. Nisbet and Fahy point to the importance of what Patterson (2013) has called 'knowledge-based journalism' to 'contextualize and critically evaluate expert knowledge, facilitate discussion that bridges entrenched ideological divisions, and promote consideration of a broader menu of policy options and technologies' (Nisbet and Fahy 2015, p. 224). Science writing and science journalism may then serve as one strategy to bring public attention and debate to evidentiary matters, although there have been concerns raised about the fall in relevance of science journalists in recent years. Dunwoody (2014), for example, argues that the shift to the digital age has undermined the roles or perceived need of science writers noting that weekly science sections of US newspapers numbered 95 in 1989, but fell to only 19 by 2013.

However, in contrast to the fall in science writing, there has been a trend in the opposite direction for the proliferation of fact-checking projects. Such efforts typically subject the claims of politicians to scrutiny and, in doing so, can highlight cases of biased uses of evidence (Graves, Nyhan and Reifler 2016). Some of these projects are linked to academic or independent institutions (e.g. www.factcheck.org), but many are now integral parts of major news outlets, such as the *New York Times* and Germany's *Der Spiegel* (Silverman 2010). One fact-checking initiative, PolitiFact of the *Tampa Bay Times* (and formerly the *St Petersburg Times*) was even awarded a Pulitzer Prize for its efforts in highlighting errors of fact in the 2008 US presidential election (Weiss 2010). However, the effectiveness of these efforts may depend on a number of factors, including the level of public understanding of policy-relevant information, as well as the political implications of having been identified as making misleading statements. Nyhan and Reifler, for example, have undertaken experiments which have found that providing lay-persons with corrections to political misstatements did not seem to reduce misconceptions (Nyhan and Reifler 2010 – see also Lewandowsky et al. 2012), but informing politicians that their work will be fact-checked did reduce the incidence of misstatements in the first place (Nyhan and Reifler 2014).

In all these ways, then, non-state institutions can supplement institutional efforts within government advisory systems to overcome bias: by serving as expert authorities on evidence, by synthesising evidence and by checking or highlighting cases when evidence is misused. Table 8.1 (see next pages) provides a summary of the various governmental and non-governmental arrangements discussed above, linking them to many of the specific manifestations of bias mentioned throughout this book. This can in no way serve as a comprehensive list of institutional forms that can address bias, but instead aims to provide an indication of the wide range of structures, rules or norms that may be considered in different settings.

Institutions govern the use of evidence

As noted earlier, a focus on the institutionalisation of bias mitigation efforts such as these can help to overcome the limitations of many past efforts in the EBP movement that have targeted individuals alone. Yet merely working to address a specific form of evidentiary bias may raise other challenges if our ultimate goal remains to improve the use of evidence in policymaking more broadly. This is, of course, because there are multiple principles that are at stake when we consider evidence use in political processes, as discussed throughout this book, and, as such, reducing bias in any one way cannot be promoted to the exclusion of all other values.

The rules and norms built into the institutions affecting evidence use will end up determining a large number of outcomes beyond simply if bias occurs. Evidence systems will decide things such as: who has the right to speak on expert matters; when and for which sorts of decisions evidence will be invoked; where budgets will be utilised to generate new evidence; and, ultimately, whose interests are represented and promoted from the operation of the evidence advisory system. In these ways, we can therefore state that such institutions work to *govern* the use of evidence in policymaking. However, understanding this leads to the recognition that governments looking to make changes to their evidence advisory systems, or civil society and expert bodies wishing to improve evidence use, will need to consider more than simply which strategies can minimise particular forms of bias. Instead, there is a need to engage with the question of what the *good governance of evidence* might look like, which requires an *explicitly normative* framework that can integrate the multiple principles and values held to be important for evidence use in the policy arena.

Governance and good governance of evidence

While there are many definitions of 'governance' in the policy studies literature (cf. Bevir 2008), here we utilise the term in a broad sense as capturing the

Table 8.1 Forms of bias and example institutional responses

Source of political evidentiary bias (see multiple politics of evidence framework in Chapter 3)	*Examples of bias*	*Illustrative cases mentioned in text*	*Example governmental responses*	*Example non-governmental responses*
Creation of evidence	Strategic design or manipulation of studies to achieve desired outcome (technical bias).	• Tobacco or pharmaceutical industry strategically designing or altering studies (Chapter 3). • Public officials manipulating data or cheating in evaluations (Chapter 4). • Reclassification of hunger data before target date to show success (Chapter 4). • Scientists' admissions of modifying results (Chapter 3).	• Delegate evaluations to arm's-length bodies (e.g. Mexico's CONEVAL). • Establish evidence advisory watchdogs within ministries (e.g. chief scientific advisors). • Create rules preventing self-evaluation of public agencies.	• Programmes that independently re-analyse trials (e.g. Oxford University's COMPare project). • Mandating conflict of interests declarations in publications. • Academic peer review practices. • Journalistic practices to question conflicts of interest.
	Choice of research topic imposes de facto policy priority (issue bias).	• Neglect of particular issues or populations in research created, e.g. neglected tropical diseases or hidden populations (Chapter 3).	• Require explicit justification for the choice of research topic in reference to other needs (for a specific policy choice). • Make policy priorities explicit and justified on policy goals (e.g. within a departmental strategy).	• Consensus statements on research priorities for fields of scientific inquiry. • Identification of neglected research areas by expert bodies.

(continued)

Table 8.1 (continued)

Source of political evidentiary bias (see multiple politics of evidence framework in Chapter 3)	*Examples of bias*	*Illustrative cases mentioned in text*	*Example governmental responses*	*Example non-governmental responses*
	Obfuscation of values within the selection of evaluation criteria (issue bias).	• Programme evaluations that do not measure concerns of all political stakeholders, e.g. harm reduction evaluations that only measure public health concerns or the choice of outcomes used to evaluate 'development' efforts (Chapters 3 and 6).	• Mandating public consultation on outcomes of policy evaluations before they are finalised.	• Establish good practices for evaluations to make the political implications of selected outcomes more explicit.
Selection of evidence	Cherry-picking of data that supports a desired conclusion (technical bias).	• Climate change arguments using limited pieces of data to exaggerate or deny trends (Chapter 3). • Selection of evidence to make the case for war (Chapter 1).	• Establishing formal bodies to systematically review evidence (e.g. NICE in the UK, Norwegian Centre for Education). • Use of expert committees and technical working groups. • Chief scientific advisor oversight. • Transparency through mechanisms such as freedom of information laws or regular public disclosures of decisions.	• Establishing expert guidelines on systematic reviews (e.g. Cochrane Collaboration guidelines). • Independent knowledge brokers or think tanks that promote best practices of evidence synthesis. • Academic bodies serving as repositories of evidence (e.g. McMaster University hosting http://www.health systems evidence.org). • Media/journalist training in science reporting and concepts of rigour and systematic review.

	Selecting evidence on a limited number of relevant concerns (issue bias).	• Gun control debates have many possible outcomes – accidental death, crime prevention, crime severity, etc. (Chapters 3 and 4). • Researchers incentivised to promote the 'policy impact' of their specific finding or topic (Chapter 4). • 'Evidence-based advocacy' (Chapter 4).	• Ensure deliberation and public representation in process to ensure all relevant outcomes are identified. • Mandate making multiple relevant outcomes explicit (e.g. akin to the strategies of multi-criteria decision analysis). • Avoid funding research based on 'impact' in terms of policy influence.	• Develop best practices on evidence synthesis that include goal clarification. • Facilitate, test or provide examples of effective deliberative processes (e.g. university deliberative democracy projects).
Interpretation of evidence	Errors from cognitive processes – e.g. thinking fast, judgement under uncertainty (technical bias).	• Incorrect causal statements, e.g. about causes of HIV decline or divers of HIV risk (Chapters 3 and 5). • Confusion over relative risk and absolute risk (Chapter 3). • Motivated reasoning leading to strategic interpretation based on position of affinity group (Chapter 5).	• Establishing procedures to double check data or to require a counter argument to be presented before final decision (e.g. 'alternative analysis' techniques). • Establish deliberative spaces that reduce polarisation or permit compromise solutions to be considered.	• Expert body self-reflection and identification of own bias (e.g. the World Bank's study of bias in its experts). • Norms to expect journalists to specify or explain risk statistics (e.g. to distinguish between absolute and relative risk). • Broader social learning to identify cognitive biases.

(continued)

Table 8.1 (continued)

Source of political evidentiary bias (see multiple politics of evidence framework in Chapter 3)	*Examples of bias*	*Illustrative cases mentioned in text*	*Example governmental responses*	*Example non-governmental responses*
	Undermining science/ denialism (technical bias).	• Climate change denial (Chapter 1), tobacco harm denial (Chapters 3 and 4) and other sowing of scientific doubt.	• Utilise independent expert bodies or agencies to evaluate evidence.	• Developing consensus positions on issues (e.g. the joint National Academies statement on climate change). • Expert statements and clarity on 'proof' versus 'evidence', and 'theory' versus 'hypothesis'.
	Interpretation of particular forms of evidence as 'best' based on method alone (issue bias).	• Using hierarchies of evidence or randomised trials to prioritise policy choices without consideration of when this is appropriate (Chapters 2, 3 and 6).	• Establish procedures to identify the appropriate evidence needed for policy concerns.	• Develop more nuanced or alternative hierarchies to judge multiple evidence types. • Avoid use of under-specified language (e.g. referring to one form of evidence as a 'gold standard'). • Broader clarity on distinguishing methods of research from values addressed.

'art of governing' (Enroth 2014), referring to the multiple arrangements and processes by which collective decisions are made and outcomes are reached in a particular context (Chhotray and Stoker 2009). This definition can be applied across a range of issues, of course – be it corporate management in the private sector, political representation in the public sector or, indeed, the arrangements governing the operation of non-human systems such as the internet. Therefore, it can also be used to capture the arrangements governing the use of evidence and further permits a direct engagement with the concept of *good governance*, which captures the normative principles held to be important within a set of governing arrangements.

The term 'good governance' has also been used in a range of settings, and the choice of elements within any definition of the term will typically reflect its particular context. In corporate settings, for instance, the term can capture concerns over behaviour of the management or board of directors of corporations (Aguilera and Cuervo-Cazurra 2009). In the international development literature, on the other hand, there has been particularly widespread engagement with the concept, using the term more directly to consider the interests of the public (Chhotray and Stoker 2009). So, for example, the United Nations Development Programme (UNDP) has specifically equated 'good governance' with 'democratic governance', which is said to be captured by systems being 'capable, responsive, inclusive, and transparent' (Clark 2011). The UN Economic and Social Commission for Asia and the Pacific, on the other hand, defines good governance as being 'participatory, consensus oriented, accountable, transparent, responsive, effective and efficient, equitable and inclusive and follows the rule of law' (2014). Meanwhile, the World Bank identified three elements in an early definition of the concept of good governance: '(i) the form of the political regime . . . (ii) the process by which authority is exercised in the management of a country's economic and social resources; and (iii) the capacity of government to design, formulate and implement policies, and, in general, to discharge government functions' (1991, p. 23). This last definition reflects a much greater focus on economic management and the achievement of desired outcomes, no doubt influenced by the World Bank's historical concern with macroeconomic growth and stability.

In general, the principles included in lists of good governance criteria can be seen to fall into two categories: those addressing the outcomes of decision making (e.g. the effectiveness or efficiency of decision making) and those speaking to the processes of decision making (e.g. accountability, transparency and adherence to the rules of law). Thinking about the good governance *of evidence* therefore requires identifying the set of values dealing with both processes and outcomes that are of particular relevance to the use of evidence within a political process. Good governance is inherently a normative concept, and this book began with two particular broad overarching normative concerns of advocates of EBP and their critics: one to do with fidelity to science and the other to do with democratic representation. However, through the course of this book, these concepts have been explored in greater depth, with additional elements discussed. This final section therefore integrates the multiple normative principles identified so far into an overarching framework of the good governance of evidence – a framework that can in particular be used to guide institutional changes aiming to improve the use of evidence in policymaking.

A framework for the good governance of evidence

This section builds on an earlier paper published jointly with a colleague (Hawkins and Parkhurst 2015) that similarly considered how elements of 'good governance' could be applied more specifically to thinking about evidence use in health policymaking. It identified four components in particular:

- The need to consider *appropriate* evidence – defined as addressing the multiple political considerations relevant to a policy decision.
- The need for *accountability* in evidence use – to ensure that the use of evidence reaches back to citizens.
- The need for *transparency* – in order to open evidence utilisation to scrutiny.
- The need for *contestability* – in the form of appeals processes and opportunity for public debate, based on the principle that having data and arguments open to questioning and challenge is a key element of the scientific process (Hawkins and Parkhurst 2015).

Many of these ideas have been addressed so far in earlier chapters of this book. Obviously, the idea of *appropriate* evidence mirrors the discussion in Chapter 6, although that chapter undertakes greater elaboration of the concept, going beyond the idea of evidence that is relevant to multiple concerns, and adding additional reflection on how evidence needs to be constructed in policy-useful ways and applicable in a local setting. The element of *accountability* is similarly reflected in multiple points made in Chapter 7 about democratic representation in the evidence advisory system. The first such point was that evidence advisory systems should be designed by actors who have an official public mandate (taking a *stewardship role*) and second was reflection on the need for final decision authority to rest with individuals who are *representative* of (and accountable to) the public. *Transparency* was similarly captured in the discussions of Chapter 7, which also explored the importance of direct public *deliberation* to ensure that public values are well represented in highly technical decision processes. The idea of *contestability* was not directly discussed in earlier chapters, but it can be seen as falling into the broader concern over adherence to scientific best practices, given the importance of peer critique and replicability in scientific pursuits. Other related scientific practices explored more directly in this book include discussions of *rigorous* (or systematic) uses of evidence and the need to use evidence judged to be of high *quality* (depending on the relevant methods to address the problems).

With these ideas in mind, we can therefore construct an expanded framework to capture eight key principles seen as constituting a good governance of evidence. These elements are described in Table 8.2 below and are graphically illustrated in Figure 8.1.

Table 8.2 Features of the good governance of evidence

Concept	*Definition and explanation*	*Example approaches*
Appropriateness	The choice of evidence follows an initial assessment of the needs of the policy decision at hand. In particular: • evidence should be selected to address the (multiple) relevant social concerns; • evidence should be considered as to whether it has been created in ways that are useful to achieve policy goals; • the applicability of the evidence to the local context should be explicitly considered.	Requiring 'goal clarification', or applying methods akin to those of multi-criteria decision analysis, which requires an initial statement of the relevant decision criteria and an attempt to prioritise different considerations. Critical questioning of evidence sources in terms of their relevance and use. Distinguishing between internal and external validity of evidence; requiring assessments of local applicability before utilisation.
Quality	The pieces of evidence used should be judged on their quality, but quality criteria should reflect the methodological principles pertaining to the form of research utilised (e.g. qualitative interviews versus clinical trials) and the nature of the data generated (e.g. descriptions versus measurements versus estimates).	Application of evidence quality criteria, with the choice of criteria based on the type of research being considered. If intervention effect is important, then existing hierarchies of evidence may be useful. If public attitudes matter, then surveys can be judged based on sample size, for instance. Similarly, a concern with future costs might employ methods such as economic modelling, with its own relevant quality criteria.
Rigour	Evidence brought to policy consideration should be rigorously (comprehensively) gathered or synthesised, avoiding selective cherry-picking.	Following good practices of systematic review, rapid review, realist review and other synthesis methods. Providing sufficient independence to evidence advisory bodies.
Stewardship	The agent setting the rules and shape of official evidence advisory systems should have a formal mandate.	Ensuring that it is authorised agents who design or alter government evidence advisory systems. Ensuring accountability to the public by those stewards shaping institutional arrangements. Resisting the imposition of institutional structures by those without a public mandate or accountability.

(continued)

Table 8.2 (continued)

Concept	*Definition and explanation*	*Example approaches*
Representation	The final decision authority for policies informed by evidence lies with democratically representative and publicly accountable officials.	Maintaining decision authority in public representatives or providing legislatures and representatives with a means to veto or over-ride technical agencies when necessary.
Transparency	Open information and clear ways for the public to see how the evidence bases informing a decision are identified and utilised.	Potentially achieved through a variety of mechanisms, including holding meetings that are open to the public, publishing transcripts of expert body deliberations, establishing freedom of information laws, etc.
Deliberation	Engagement with the public in ways that enable multiple competing values and concerns to be considered in the policy process and to give attention to different points of view, even if not all concerns can be selected in the final policy decision (cf. Fishkin and Luskin 2005; Gutmann and Thompson 2009).	Direct public consultations over issues can also be supplemented with a variety of formalised deliberative mechanisms such as citizens juries, citizens panels, planning cells, consensus conferences, etc. (cf. Abelson et al. 2001; Fishkin 2009; Papadopoulos and Warin 2007).
Contestability	Having technical evidence and scientific research used in policy decisions that are open to critical questioning and appeal. This can involve challenging particular scientific findings, but also enables challenges over decisions about which evidence to utilise (e.g. to question the appropriateness of the evidence for a specific case).	Establishing formal appeals procedures and rules for decisions of evidence-synthesising bodies. Subjecting expert conclusions to peer review or scrutiny.

Source: Adapted from Hawkins and Parkhurst (2015).

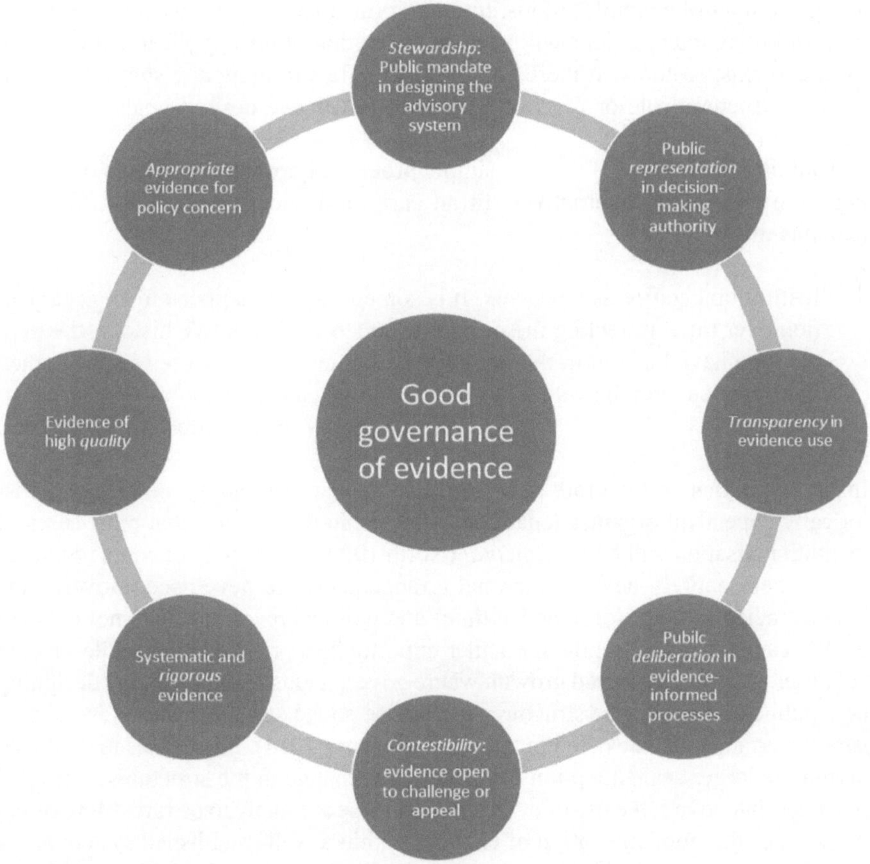

Figure 8.1 Elements of the good governance of evidence.

Taken in combination, this framework ultimately reflects a view that rigorous, relevant and unbiased pieces of evidence should be used to inform policy decisions that remain representative of, and accountable to, local populations.

Achieving the good governance of evidence through a process of guided evolution

The good governance of evidence framework assembles the multiple principles and concerns addressed throughout this book into a structure to inform processes of institution building that aim to improve the use of evidence in policymaking. It is of course quite intuitive when pursuing a goal to ask the question of 'what works' to get there, and some may directly ask which institutional structures indeed 'work' to achieve the good governance of evidence. However, Chapter 2's caveats about seeking 'what works' out of context remain pertinent. Table 8.1 of course provides a large number of examples of institutional forms that prove informative. But, just as most policy interventions will need consideration of how applicable they are to local contexts, so too will there be a need to reflect on how any suggested institutional structure, rule or practice will work to achieve desired goals when it is adopted in a local setting.

Building institutions is rarely a simple process of copying templates or choosing from a menu of alternatives. In an early and widely cited work, Selznick explains that:

> Institutionalization is a *process*. It is something that happens to an organization over time, reflecting the organization's own distinctive history, the people who have been in it, the groups it embodies and the vested interests they have created, and the way it has adapted to its environment.
>
> (1957, p. 16, emphasis in original)

Institutional change therefore necessarily takes place within an existing and historically dependent organisational context. This, in turn, means that most cases of institutionalisation will be *incremental* (North 1990). There may of course be some cases where entirely new institutional arrangements are developed. Government bureaucracies do get re-designed at times and political revolutions are not unheard of. We can also recognise the particular opportunities presented in middle-income countries experiencing rapid growth, where governments may be quickly designing new public administrative structures to provide social services where few administrative arrangements existed in the past (Ginsburg 2014). Such cases may indeed permit the larger-scale adoption of institutional change in the structures, rules and practices that govern the use of evidence. Yet these are likely to be rare. More often, we will see the implementation of changes within a well-established system and a need for institutions to adapt their functions and values in line with existing political arrangements. Indeed, while Colombia's IETS programme was explicitly modelled on NICE in the UK, as noted earlier, the agency is located in a different administrative position from NICE, undertaking slightly different functions and roles, with subsequent implications for how much it can (or cannot) influence health policy decision making and health service provision (Castro 2014).

Selznick (1957) is also widely recognised for describing institutionalisation as including the processes by which organisations are 'infused with values' – values that go beyond their operational requirements and instead link to their broader goals (von Maravić and Dudek 2013). However, if the broader goal is to build institutions to *improve* the use of evidence, we must directly address this question of what principles we use to judge improvement and which values to therefore infuse. The good governance of evidence framework provides us with just such a normative template that can inform this thinking. Taken as such, the process of institutional change to improve the use of evidence can be defined as a process of *guided evolution* – *guided* because it requires a normative set of goals to direct change efforts in line with efforts for improvement, and *evolutionary* in the way in which it incrementally shapes or alters institutional arrangements within an existing political system.[1]

It is not common to find published cases illustrating such deliberate processes of guided evolution, whereby an agency such as a government department has attempted to institutionalise improved uses of evidence in line with explicitly stated principles. But one example can be seen in the experience of the UK's Department of Environment, Food and Rural Affairs (DEFRA), which did undertake just such a process in the mid-2000s and whose experience was written up to inform the Australian aid agency's 'Knowledge Sector Initiative', which funds efforts to improve evidence use in Indonesia. The experience and approach of DEFRA is summarised in Box 8.1 below.

Box 8.1 Guided evolution to institutionalise evidence improvements: the case of DEFRA

Much of the text in this example has been summarised from Shaxson (2014)

DEFRA is the UK government department (ministry) responsible for issues such as environmental protection, agriculture, forests and marine environments, and rural services (DEFRA 2015). As described by Shaxson (2014), in 2004, the Department was responsible for a research budget of £325 million (just under US$600 million at the time) and identified a need to more systematically ensure that these funds were used to help the Department achieve its strategic priorities and goals. An internal Science Strategy Team, which had been tasked with ensuring the technical quality of the evidence base, decided to develop an 'Evidence Investment Strategy' to serve this purpose. Three particular ideas initially informed the creation of this strategy: (1) that different types of evidence from different disciplines were needed to make effective policy; (2) that there was need for a clear 'line of sight' between evidence and the Department's policy priorities and objectives; and (3) that the quality of the process of using evidence was as important as the quality of the evidence itself. DEFRA's first Evidence Investment Strategy (which ran from 2006 to 2010) was designed primarily to change how evidence budgets were allocated and managed,

(continued)

1 A similar idea comes from the field of international development in the form of 'Problem-Driven Iterative Adaption'. This approach was intended to move beyond past failures of organisational reform, which simply shifted what organisations look like, to actually change what they do in practice. The approach is said to require locally defined problem-driven approaches that occur through 'positive deviance and experimentation', which in turn facilitates experiential learning that can feedback into further experiments and changes (Andrews, Pritchett and Woolcock 2012). In these ways, this approach parallels many of the ideas of guided evolution presented here, although guided by problems rather than governance principles per se. It further speaks to the need for locally owned and demanded changes occurring from within existing institutional contexts rather than simply assuming that structures and solutions can be imported from elsewhere.

(continued)

yet undertaking the process led to critical reflection on the role of evidence within the Department as a whole. This resulted in DEFRA adopting what was described as a 'systematic approach to improving how it sources and uses evidence to inform policymaking' (Shaxson 2014, p. iii).

Louise Shaxson, who served as an advisor to the Science Strategy Team (and authored the report summarised here), explained that the goal of the Evidence Investment Strategy process was to make evidence-informed decision making 'business as usual' within DEFRA (personal communication, 29 April 2016). Doing so, however, meant explicitly identifying what an improved use of evidence would look like. A set of key principles was elucidated on which to base the initial strategy – principles that overlap with several elements of the good governance of evidence framework described in this chapter. These were described as follows:

1 A need for evidence that specifically responded to policy goals and priorities (recognising the importance of evidence challenging these goals as well).
2 Policymakers to recognise a range of different types of evidence as relevant (statistical data, stakeholder perspectives, evidence from monitoring and evaluation, etc.).
3 A balance to be struck between short-term needs and long-term priorities.
4 A commitment to re-analysis of older evidence as well as commissioning new evidence.

A fifth principle, seen as underlying all the others, was that of 'transparency in the evidence base' – specifically embraced due to a recognition of a need for 'good governance of the evidence base' so as to ensure that stakeholders were well represented and bought into the evidence-utilisation process (see Shaxson 2014, p. vii).

The first Evidence Investment Strategy was further developed in two subsequent iterations. The result has been that DEFRA has been incrementally experimenting with its institutional arrangements over time to embed its key principles and mainstream them within operational processes. So, for example, during the second strategy process (which ran from 2010 to 2013), the agency moved evidence specialists from a central directorate into different policy teams, where they held their own research budgets. However, it was soon learned that this could increase the likelihood of duplication in research efforts, so changes were made whereby the evidence specialists remained in place, but budgetary control moved back to a central body. Other changes have been seen as well, such as shifting work previously allocated to external consultants to the central evidence directorate or taking steps to increasingly link departmental business plans with evidence procurement.

DEFRA developed explicit principles concerned with evidence relevance, quality and public representation that have steered a decade of gradual administrative changes to improve evidentiary practice. In doing so, its experience provides a rare documented example of a government agency undertaking a deliberate process of *guided evolution* to institutionalise aspects of the good governance of evidence, reflecting many of the ideas described throughout this chapter.

Conclusion

In many ways, this book has followed a path that has touched on a series of normative concerns linked with conceptual discussions. In Part I, Chapters 1 and 2 introduced the EBP movement as both important and limited in key ways: important in how it embraces laudable goals such as a desire to ensure that science is used accurately with the ultimate aim to improve social outcomes, but limited in its conceptualisation of the policy process. This limitation then led to the identification of a set of challenges in evidence utilisation within policymaking. Two distinct forms of bias were identified: technical bias, reflecting a need for scientific fidelity; and issue bias, reflecting a competing concern over democratic representation. It was noted that 'improving' the use of evidence in policy with both of these in mind requires a decidedly political approach – one that recognises the realities of decision making in contested policy arenas. In Part II of the book, Chapters 3, 4 and 5 moved on to explore these biases, working to identify their forms, origins and manifestations, particularly in relation to our political values. This was undertaken based on the premise that by developing a more rigorous conceptual understanding of how these forms of bias arise, we might have greater success in mitigating or avoiding them in the future. In Part III of the book, Chapters 6 and 7 followed by undertaking further normative discussions, reconceptualising what might constitute 'good evidence for policy' (Chapter 6) and what might be judged as a 'good use of evidence' within a policy process (Chapter 7). This has then led to this final chapter, which returned to the initial question of how to improve the use of evidence in policymaking. In particular, it discussed the need to build institutional structures that help reduce bias and that serve to govern the use of evidence. This overall path taken is illustrated in Figure 8.2 below.

The direct engagement with normative concerns throughout many of the previous chapters helps to distinguish this book from several other contemporary works on evidence use that employ a policy perspective. While sharing much of the same theoretical basis and no doubt overlapping at times, other authors have particularly been concerned with describing the many meanings and manifestations of evidence 'use' (cf. Nutley, Walter and Davies 2007; Weiss 1979) or exploring the utilisation of evidence in particular policy case studies (cf. Cairney 2015; Smith 2013). Here, however, we have kept at the fore the primary question of what it means to *improve* the use of evidence in policymaking. This starting point derives from the overarching goal of the EBP movement to achieve better social outcomes, while recognising the limitations that movement has faced in applying its ideas within political settings. As noted previously, the idea of using scientific research, evidence and tools of policy analysis to help achieve social and political goals has a long history in the field of public policy (DeLeon 2006). Many see its roots in Harold Lasswell's concept of the policy sciences developed in the 1970s (DeLeon 2006; Lasswell 1970, 1971). Others have noted similar thinking in the work of John Dewey, who saw the usefulness of science in solving

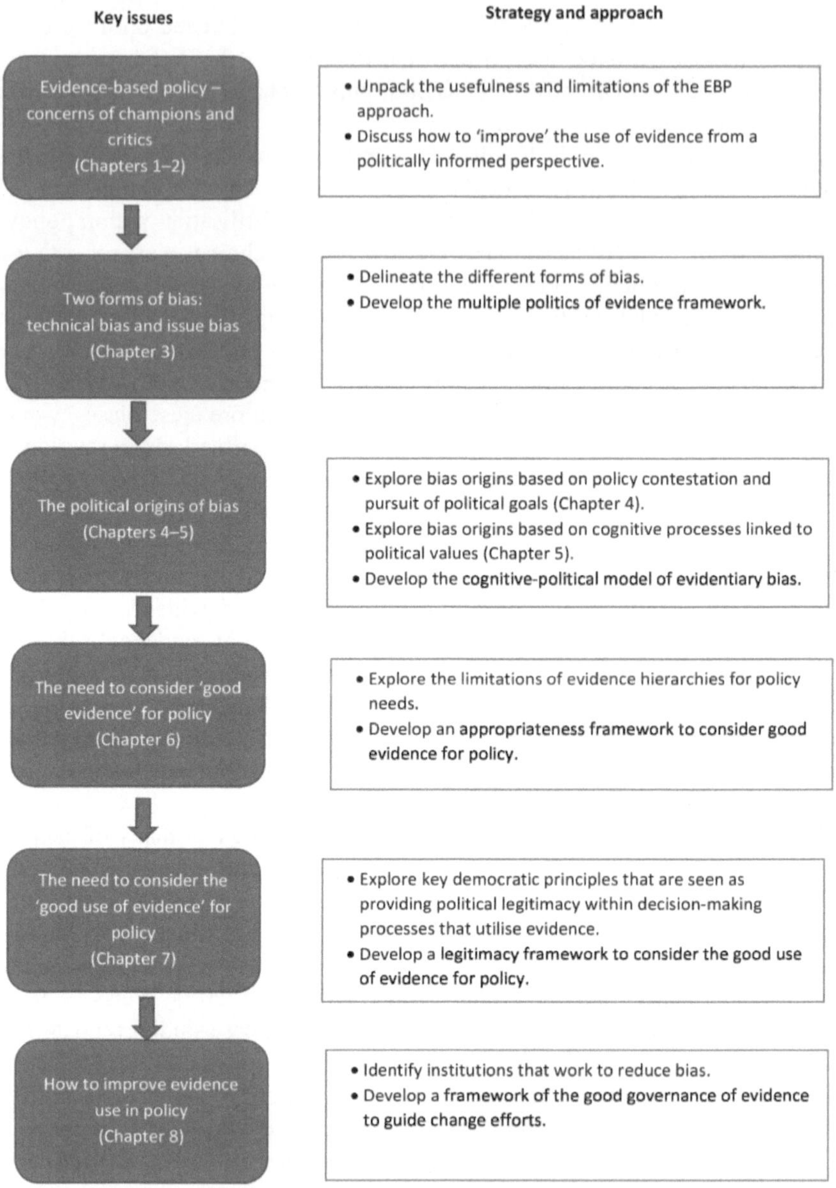

Figure 8.2 The conceptual path taken.

social problems, but who raised concerns over reductionism of policy to scientific method as early as the 1920s (Dewey 1954 [1927]; Johnston 2002). In many ways, this book has revisited these ideas, bringing their pragmatism and political orientation to the current EBP debates.

Although based around a set of normative discussions, this book makes no claim to ideological perfection or moral authority. The reader is free to agree or disagree with the values stated or implicit in any of the chapters or, indeed, within any elements of the good governance of evidence framework proposed. Yet effort has been made to avoid taking sides on the specific policy issues discussed. Instead, the book has drawn upon widely shared value positions to address the broader cross-cutting questions of evidence use. So, for example, the idea that science should be used faithfully and accurately does underlie many chapter discussions, but few would argue that incorrect, cherry-picked or misused evidence is preferable to accurate, rigorous and valid examples. Other principles embedded in the book relate more specifically to the needs and realities of policymaking, of course, over which there is no shortage of disagreement. Indeed, defining *good* evidence as based around a lens of *appropriateness* serves to establish a relative value claim. Again, though, the normative position taken in Chapter 6 is hardly controversial, arguing that *better* evidence can be judged against how well it addresses the multiple policy goals or concerns at hand (whichever they happen to be). It is much harder to justify a contrary position – that the inappropriate application of evidence to situations where it is not relevant is somehow preferable. Chapter 7 perhaps raises the biggest questions, as it starts from a basic assumption that democratic representation is an important value to pursue in political systems dealing with evidence. Some might alternatively argue that transparency or public deliberation can be justified without this – for example, because they are necessary to ensure that policy outcomes are reached effectively. However, such a view accepts democratic inclusion only in situations when it improves outcomes. The position taken in Chapter 7 goes beyond this and does so by drawing on authors who promote democratic representation in technical decision processes as an important value in and of itself. Indeed, public consultation can at times slow down decision processes or increase their costs, yet the importance of consulting the public is widely held to come from the fundamental importance of ensuring appropriate consideration of public needs and wants in political decisions.

Regardless of whether the reader agrees with each proposition, it is important to recognise why this book has been so explicitly concerned with principles of evidence use. As noted in Chapter 2, much past work coming out of the EBP movement has assumed that *more* evidence use is inherently *better* evidence use (Smith 2013). Such a belief appears to rest on an assumption that evidence works to serve a problem solving role in situations where all outcomes have been agreed. But such situations are the exception, rather than the rule, in policymaking (Weiss 1979). As such, many evidence utilisation concepts and strategies arising from this position have typically been under-specified – failing to ask *which* evidence for *what* goals in particular. The EBP community has had an explicit concern with the *politicisation of science*, yet it has generally not considered the *depoliticisation of politics* when promoting certain forms of evidence uptake – a blind spot that cannot continue to be unaddressed given the decidedly political nature of public policymaking.

The alternative approach promoted here has been to explore the key principles relevant to the realms of both evidence utilisation and political decision making.

To *improve* the use of evidence in policy requires an explicit engagement with the question of what constitutes *better* use from a political perspective. Attempting to answer this question has led to the recognition that long-term improvement requires building institutional arrangements that can address key forms of evidentiary bias while simultaneously incorporating principles of democratic representation. This involves the institutionalisation of structures, rules, processes and practices that work to ensure that rigorous, valid and relevant bodies of evidence are utilised through transparent and deliberative processes to inform decisions that ultimately remain representative of, and accountable to, local populations. Achieving this would constitute an important step towards establishing the good governance of evidence and could help to better realise the full potential of evidence to accomplish our collective social policy goals.

References

Abelson, J., P-G. Forest, J. Eyles, P. Smith, E. Martin and F.-P. Gauvin. 2001. 'Deliberations about deliberation: issues in the design and evaluation of public consultation processes'. McMaster University Centre for Health Economics and Policy Analysis Research Working Paper 01-04, June.

Aguilera, Ruth V. and Alvaro Cuervo-Cazurra. 2009. 'Codes of good governance'. *Corporate Governance: An International Review* 17(3): 376–387. doi: 10.1111/j.1467-8683.2009.00737.x.

Andrews, Matt, Lant Pritchett and Michael Woolcock. 2012. *Escaping Capability Traps through Problem-Driven Iterative Adaptation (PDIA).* Washinton DC: Center for Global Development.

Baltussen, Rob and Louis Niessen. 2006. 'Priority setting of health interventions: The need for multi-criteria decision analysis'. *Cost Effectiveness and Resource Allocation* 4(1): 14. doi: 10.1186/1478-7547-4-1.

Belton, Valerie and Theodor Stewart. 2002. *Multiple Criteria Decision Analysis: An Integrated Approach.* Boston: Kluwer Academic Publishers.

Bevir, Mark. 2008. *Key Concepts in Governance*. London: Sage.

Cairney, Paul. 2015. *The Politics of Evidence-Based Policymaking.* London: Palgrave Pivot.

Castro, Hector. 2014. 'Assessing the Feasibility of Conducting and Using Health Technology Assessment in Colombia. The case of severe haemophilia'. Doctor of Public Health thesis, London School of Hygiene and Tropical Medicine.

Castro, Manuel Fernando, Gladys Lopez-Acevedo, Gita Beker Busjeet and Ximena Fernandez Ordonez. 2009. Mexico's M&E system: scaling up from the sectoral to the national level. Washington, D.C.: World Bank.

Center for Deliberative Democracy. Undated. 'Home page'. Stanford University, http://cdd.stanford.edu, accessed 8 July 2016.

Chhotray, Vasudha and Gerry Stoker. 2009. *Governance Theory and Practice: A Cross-disciplinary Approach.* Basingstoke: Palgrave Macmillan.

Clark, Helen. 2011. 'UNDP Chief: poorest countries must have a say in shaping their future'. Fourth United Nations Conference on the Least Developed Countries: High Level Interactive Thematic Debate on Good Governance at All Levels, Istanbul, 11 May.

COMPare. 2016. 'Home page'. Nuffield Department of Primary Care Sciences, http://compare-trials.org, accessed 8 July 2016.

Cookson, Richard. 2013. 'Can the NICE "end-of-life premium" be given a coherent ethical justification?' *Journal of Health Politics, Policy and Law* 38(6): 1129–1148.

DEFRA. 2015. *Department for Environment, Food and Rural Affairs annual report and accounts: 2014–15.* London: Williams Lea Group on behalf of the Controller of Her Majesty's Stationery Office.

DeLeon, Peter. 2006. 'The historical roots of the field'. In *The Oxford Handbook of Public Policy*, edited by Michael Moran, Martin Rein and Robert E. Goodin, pp. 39–57. Oxford: Oxford University Press.

Dewey, John. 1954 (1927). *The public and its Problems*. Athens, OH: Swallow Press/Ohio University Press.

Duncan, David Ewing. 2007. 'The anti-science president'. *MIT Technology Review*, 12 July. https://www.technologyreview.com/s/408236/the-anti-science-president, accessed 11 July 2016.

Dunwoody, Sharon. 2014. 'Science journalism: Prospects in the digital age'. In *Routledge Handbook of Public Communication of Science and Technology*, 2nd edn, edited by Massimano Bucchi and Brian Trench, pp. 27–39. Abingdon: Routledge.

Enroth, Henrik. 2014. 'Governance: The art of governing after governmentality'. *European Journal of Social Theory* 17(1): 60–76. doi: 10.1177/1368431013491818.

EPPI-Centre. Undated. 'Welcome to the EPPI-Centre'. UCL: Institute of Education, http://eppi.ioe.ac.uk/cms, accessed 8 July 2016.

Fishbein, Warren and Gregory Treverton. 2004. 'Rethinking "alternative analysis" to address transnational threats'. https://www.cia.gov/library/kent-center-occasional-papers/vol3no2.htm, accessed 11 July 2016.

Fishkin, James. 2009. *When the People Speak: Deliberative Democracy and Public Consultation*. Oxford: Oxford University Press.

Fishkin, James and Robert Luskin. 2005. 'Experimenting with a democratic ideal: Deliberative polling and public opinion'. *Acta Politica* 40(3): 284–298.

Fouilleux, Eves, Jacques de Maillard and Andy Smith. 2005. 'Technical or political? The working groups of the EU Council of Ministers'. *Journal of European Public Policy* 12(4): 609–623. doi: 10.1080/13501760500160102.

Ginsburg, Tom. 2014. 'The politics of law and development in middle-income countries'. In *Law and Development of Middle-Income Countries: Avoiding the Middle-Income Trap*, edited by Randall Peerenboom and Tom Ginsburg, pp. 21–35. Cambridge: Cambridge University Press.

Godlee, Fiona. 2009. 'NICE at 10'. *British Medical Journal* 338. doi: 10.1136/bmj.b344.

Gornitzka, Åse and Ulf Sverdrup. 2008. 'Who consults? The configuration of expert groups in the European Union'. *West European Politics* 31(4): 725–750. doi: 10.1080/01402380801905991.

Graves, Lucas, Brendan Nyhan and Jason Reifler. 2016. 'Understanding innovations in journalistic practice: A field experiment examining motivations for fact-checking'. *Journal of Communication* 66(1): 102–138. doi: 10.1111/jcom.12198.

Gutmann, Amy and Dennis Thompson. 2009. *Why Deliberative Democracy?* Princeton: Princeton University Press.

Halligan, John. 1995. 'Policy advice and the public service'. In *Governance in a Changing Environment*, edited by Guy Peters and Donald Savoie, pp. 138–172. Montreal: Canadian Centre for Management Development.

Hawkins, Benjamin and Justin Parkhurst. 2015. 'The "good governance" of evidence in health policy'. *Evidence & Policy: A Journal of Research, Debate and Practice*. doi: 10.1332/174426415X14430058455412.

Johnston, James Scott. 2002. 'John Dewey and the role of scientific method in aesthetic experience'. *Studies in Philosophy and Education* 21(1): 1–15.

Joint Academies of Science. Undated. 'Joint science academies' statement: Global response to climate change', http://nationalacademies.org/onpi/06072005.pdf, accessed 8 July 2016.

Knowledge Centre for Education. 2015. 'About the Knowledge Centre for Education'. Research Council of Norway, http://www.forskningsradet.no/prognett-kunnskaps-senter/About_the_Knowledge_Centre/1254009289413?lang=en, accessed 8 July 2016.

Koon, Adam, Devaki Nambiar and Krishna Rao. 2012. 'Embedding of research into decision-making processes'. Alliance for Health Policy and Systems Research and Public Health Foundation of India. http://www.who.int/alliance-hpsr/alliancehpsr_back groundpaperembeddingresearch.pdf, accessed 11 July 2016.

Koon, Adam, Krishna Rao, Nhan Tran and Abdul Ghaffar. 2013. 'Embedding health policy and systems research into decision-making processes in low-and middle-income countries'. *Health Research Policy and Systems* 11(1): 30. doi: 10.1186/1478-4505-11-30.

Lasswell, Harold. 1970. 'The emerging conception of the policy sciences'. *Policy Sciences* 1(1): 3–14.

——. 1971. *A Pre-view of Policy Sciences.* New York: Elsevier.

Lavis, John, Govin Permanand, Cristina Catallo and BRIDGE Study Team. 2013. *How Can Knowledge Brokering Be Advanced in a Country's Health System?* Copenhagen: WHO Regional Office for Europe.

Lewandowsky, Stephan, Ullrich K. H. Ecker, Colleen M. Seifert, Norbert Schwartz and John Cook. 2012. 'Misinformation and its correction continued influence and successful debiasing'. *Psychological Science in the Public Interest* 13(3): 106–131.

Lopez, Blanca Lila Gracia. 2012. 'Mexico: A social protection floor'. In *Sharing Innovative Experiences: Successful Social Protection Floor Experiences*, edited by UNDP, pp. 291–311. New York: Special Unit for South-South Cooperation, UNDP.

Lowndes, Vivien and Mark Roberts. 2013. *Why Institutions Matter.* Basingstoke: Palgrave Macmillan.

Makerere University College of Health Sciences. Undated. 'Makerere University College of Health Sciences reaches out to policymakers for research evidence needs'. http://chs.mak.ac.ug/content/makerere-university-college-health-sciences-reaches-out-policy-makers-research-evidence-need, accessed 8 July 2016.

March, James G. and Johan P. Olsen. 1984. 'The new institutionalism: Organizational factors in political life'. *American Political Science Review* 78(3): 734–749. doi: 10.2307/1961840.

——. 2006. 'The logic of appropriateness'. In *The Oxford Handbook of Public Policy*, edited by Michael Moran, Martin Rein and Robert Goodin, pp. 689–708. Oxford: Oxford University Press.

McMaster Health Forum. Undated. 'McMaster Health Forum'. McMaster University, https://www.mcmasterhealthforum.org, accessed 8 July 2016.

Mendizabal, Enrique and Kristen Sample. 2009. *Thinking Politics: Think Tanks and Political Parties in Latin America.* London: Overseas Development Institute.

National Academies of Sciences, Engineering and Medicine. 2016. 'Publications'. http://www.nationalacademies.org/publications/index.html, accessed 8 July 2016.

NICE. 2013. *NICE Charter.* London: National Institute for Health and Care Excellence,.

NICE International. 2011. *NICE International Review 2011.* London: National Institute for Health and Clinical Excellence.

Nisbet, Matthew and Declan Fahy. 2015. 'The need for knowledge-based journalism in politicized science debates'. *Annals of the American Academy of Political and Social Science* 658(1): 223–234. doi: 10.1177/0002716214559887.

North, Douglass. 1990. *Institutions, Institutional Change and Economic Performance*. Cambridge: Cambridge University Press.

Nutley, Sandra, Isabel Walter and Nick Bland. 2002. 'The institutional arrangements for connecting evidence and policy: The case of drug misuse'. *Public Policy and Administration* 17(3): 76–94.

Nutley, Sandra, Isabel Walter and Huw Davies. 2007. *Using Evidence: How Research Can Inform Public Services*. Bristol: Policy Press.

Nyhan, Brendan and Jason Reifler. 2010. 'When corrections fail: The persistence of political misperceptions'. *Political Behavior* 32(2): 303–330. doi: 10.1007/s11109-010-9112-2.

——. 2014. 'The effect of fact-checking on elites: A field experiment on U.S. state legislators'. *American Journal of Political Science* 59(3): 628–640. doi: 10.1111/ajps.12162.

Papadopoulos, Yannis and Philippe Warin. 2007. 'Are innovative, participatory and deliberative procedures in policy making democratic and effective?' *European Journal of Political Research* 46(4): 445–472. doi: 10.1111/j.1475-6765.2007.00696.x.

Patterson, Thomas. 2013. *Informing the News: The Need for Knowledge-Based Journalism*. New York: Vintage Books.

Peters, Guy. 2005. *Institutional Theory in Political Science*. London: Continuum.

Pew Research Center. 2016. 'About Pew Research Center', http://www.pewresearch.org/about, accessed 11 July 2016.

Program for Deliberative Democracy. 2005. 'Home page'. http://hss.cmu.edu/pdd, accessed 11 JUyl 2016.

Selznick, Philip. 1957. *Leadership in Administration: A Sociological Interpretation*. Berkeley: University of California Press.

Shaxson, Louise. 2014. *Investing in Evidence: Lessons from the UK Department for Environment, Food and Rural Affairs*. Kementerian PPN/Bappenas and Australian Aid Knowledge Sector Initiative.

Silverman, Graig. 2010. 'Inside the world's largest fact checking operation'. *Columbia Journalism Review*, 9 April.

Silverman, Rosa. 2013. 'Homeopathy is "rubbish", says chief medical officer'. *The Telegraph*, 24 January, http://www.telegraph.co.uk/news/health/news/9822744/Homeopathy-is-rubbish-says-chief-medical-officer.html, accessed 8 July 2016.

Smith, James. 1991. *Idea Brokers: Think Tanks and the Rise of the New Policy Elite*. New York: Free Press.

Smith, Katherine. 2013. *Beyond Evidence-Based Policy in Public Health: The Interplay of Ideas*. Basingstoke: Palgrave Macmillan.

Sorenson, Corinna, Michael Drummond, Panos Kanavos and Alistair McGuire. 2008. *National Institute for Health and Clinical Excellence (NICE). How Does it Work and What are the Implications for the US?* Washington DC: National Pharmaceutical Council.

Starr, Mark, Iain Chalmers, Mike Clarke and Andrew Oxman. 2009. 'The origins, evolution, and future of the Cochrane Database of Systematic Reviews'. *International Journal of Technology Assessment in Health Care* 51(1): 182–195.

UK Government. 2013. *What Works: Evidence Centres for Social Policy*. London: UK Cabinet Office.

United Nations Economic and Social Commission for Asia and the Pacific. 2014. 'What is good governance?', http://www.unescap.org/pdd/prs/ProjectActivities/Ongoing/gg/governance.asp, accessed 8 July 2016.

Van Kammen, Jessika, Don de Savigny and Nelson Sewankambo. 2006. 'Using knowledge brokering to promote evidence-based policy-making: The need for support structures'. *Bulletin of the World Health Organization* 84: 608–612.

Von Maravić, Patrick and Sonja Dudek. 2013. 'Representative bureaucracy in Germany? From passive to active intercultural opening'. In *Representative Bureaucracy in Action: Country Profiles from the Americas, Europe, Africa and Asia*, edited by Patrick von Maravić, Guy Peters and Eckhard Schröter, pp. 99–110. Cheltenham: Edward Elgar.

Weiss, Carol H. 1979. 'The many meanings of research utilization'. *Public Administration Review* 39(5): 426–431.

Weiss, Daniel. 2010. 'Truth in advertising'. *Campaigns & Elections* 32(298): 34–37.

World Bank. 1991. *Managing Development: The Governance Dimension.* Washington DC: World Bank.

Index

Page numbers followed by an italicised *n*, *b*, *t* or *f* refer to notes, boxes, tables or figures respectively.